PILATE FOR SENIORS OVER 60

The Ultimate Guide to Staying Fit and Healthy in Your Senior Years

ALISTAIR PROSE

To my Grandfather, you inspire me greatly

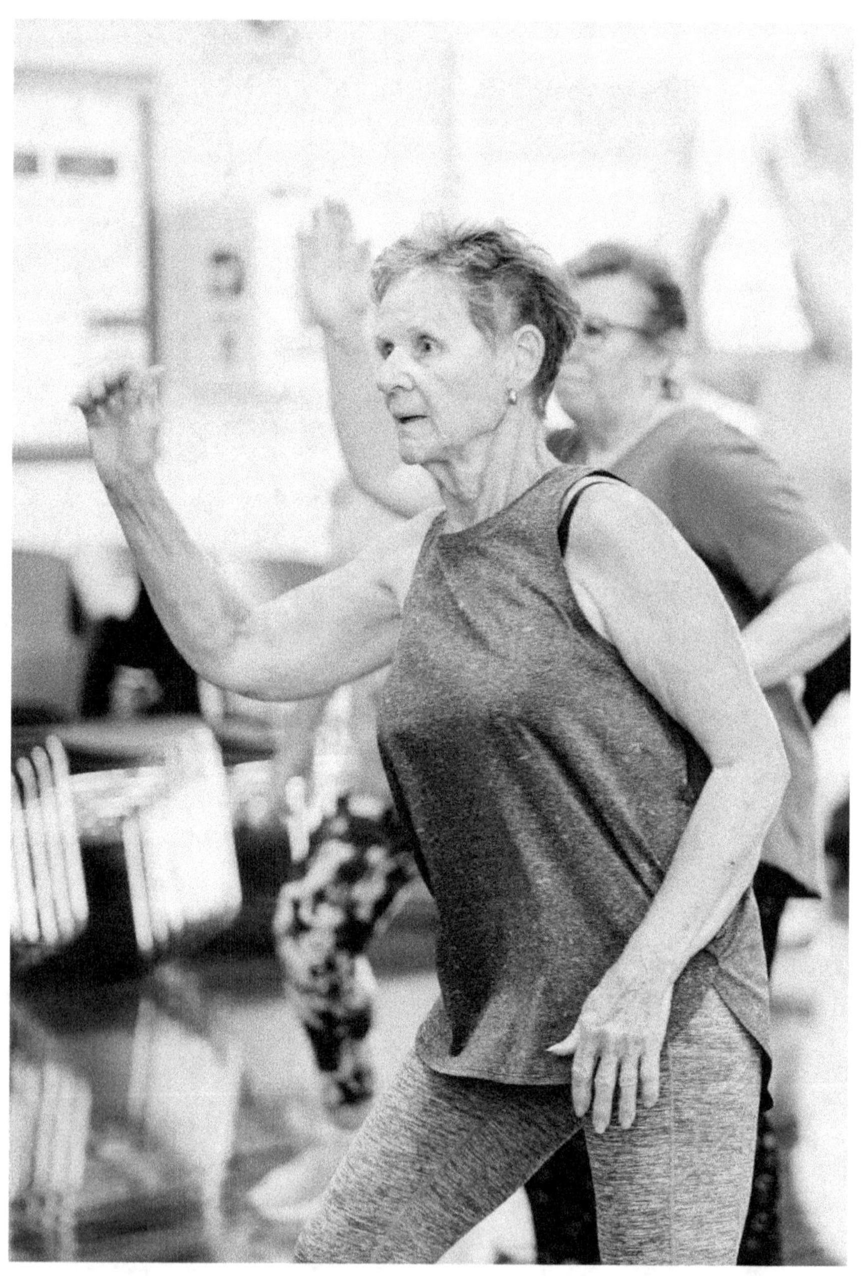

<u>FORWARD</u>

Welcome to the world of Pilates! As we age, it becomes increasingly important to take care of our bodies and maintain our mobility, flexibility, and strength. Pilates is a wonderful form of exercise that can help seniors over 60 achieve these goals and more.

Pilates focuses on building a strong core, improving posture, and developing long, lean muscles. It is a low-impact exercise that is gentle on the joints, making it a perfect choice for seniors who may have some limitations or injuries. In addition to physical benefits, Pilates can also improve mental health by reducing stress, increasing focus and concentration, and promoting a sense of overall well-being.

In this book, you will find a comprehensive guide to Pilates for seniors over 60. Whether you are new to Pilates or have been practising for years, this book will help you deepen your understanding of the practice and its benefits. You will learn about the foundational principles of Pilates, including breathing, alignment, and control. You will also find a variety of exercises and routines tailored specifically to the needs of seniors, with modifications and adaptations for different levels of ability.

Pilates is a practice that can be enjoyed at any age, and it is never too late to start. With the help of this book, you can begin or continue your Pilates journey with confidence, knowing that you are taking a positive step towards improving your health and well-being. So grab your mat, put on some comfortable clothes, and let's get started!

Table of Contents

CHAPTER 1:

Introduction to Pilates for Seniors

Pilates is a popular form of exercise that has grown in popularity in recent years, and for good reason. It is a low-impact workout that emphasizes strength, flexibility, and balance. This makes it an excellent option for seniors who want to remain active and healthy.

Our bodies change as we age, making it more difficult to engage in physical activities. This can result in a loss of strength, flexibility, and balance, increasing the risk of falls and injuries. Pilates is an excellent exercise for seniors because it can help with these important aspects of physical fitness.

Pilates is a low-impact workout, which is one of its many benefits. This means it is gentle on the joints and lowers the risk of injury. Many of the exercises are also done on the mat, making it suitable for people of all fitness levels.

Pilates promotes mindfulness and relaxation in addition to physical benefits. Stress and anxiety can be reduced by focusing on proper breathing and posture, which is especially important for seniors who may be dealing with chronic health conditions or other challenges.

Pilates is an excellent choice for seniors looking for a safe and effective form of exercise. By incorporating Pilates into your routine, you can improve your overall physical fitness, reduce your risk of falls and injuries, and promote a sense of well-being and relaxation. So why not give it a shot and see what it can do for you?

The benefits of Pilates for seniors

Pilates is a form of exercise that focuses on developing core strength, balance, flexibility, and posture. It has become increasingly popular among people of all ages, but it is particularly beneficial for seniors. In this article, we will explore the many benefits of Pilates for seniors.

Improved Core Strength

One of the main benefits of Pilates for seniors is improved core strength. The core muscles include the abdominals, back, and pelvic floor muscles. These muscles play a vital role in supporting the spine and maintaining good posture. As we age, our core muscles can weaken, which can lead to poor posture, back pain, and other health issues.

Pilates exercises are designed to strengthen the core muscles by focusing on movements that engage the abdominals and back muscles. This can help seniors to maintain good posture, reduce back pain, and improve overall mobility.

Increased Flexibility

Another key benefit of Pilates for seniors is increased flexibility. As we age, our muscles and joints can become stiff and inflexible, which can limit our range of motion and make it difficult to perform everyday activities. Pilates exercises are designed to improve flexibility by focusing on controlled movements that stretch and lengthen the muscles. This can help seniors to maintain a full range of motion, reduce the risk of injury, and improve overall mobility.

Improved Balance and Stability

Maintaining good balance and stability is essential for seniors, as it can help to prevent falls and injuries. Pilates exercises are designed to improve balance and stability by focusing on movements that challenge the body's ability to maintain equilibrium.

Pilates exercises that involve standing on one leg or balancing on an unstable surface can help to improve balance and stability. This can help seniors to feel more confident in their ability to perform everyday activities and reduce their risk of falls and injuries.

Reduced Joint Pain

Many seniors suffer from joint pain, particularly in the knees, hips, and back. Pilates exercises are designed to be low-impact, which makes them an ideal form of exercise for seniors who want to stay active without aggravating joint pain.

Pilates exercises that focus on stretching and strengthening the muscles around the joints can help to reduce joint pain and improve mobility. This can help seniors to perform everyday activities with less pain and discomfort.

Improved Posture

Good posture is essential for maintaining good health as we age. Poor posture can lead to back pain, neck pain, and other health issues. Pilates exercises are designed to improve posture by focusing on movements that strengthen the core muscles and align the spine.

Pilates exercises that focus on proper alignment and posture can help seniors to maintain good posture, reduce back pain, and improve overall mobility.

Reduced Stress and Anxiety

Many seniors deal with chronic health conditions, such as arthritis or heart disease, which can be stressful and anxiety-provoking. Pilates exercises are designed to promote relaxation and reduce stress and anxiety.

Pilates exercises that focus on proper breathing and relaxation can help seniors to feel calmer and more centered. This can improve overall well-being and help seniors to better cope with the stressors of daily life.

Increased Energy and Stamina

As we age, we may experience a decline in energy and stamina, which can make it difficult to perform everyday activities. Pilates exercises are designed to improve energy and stamina by increasing cardiovascular endurance and improving muscle strength and flexibility.

Pilates exercises that involve movement and cardiovascular activity can help seniors to feel more energized and improve overall endurance. This can make it easier to perform everyday activities and maintain a higher level of activity and independence.

Improved Quality of Life

Perhaps the most important benefit of Pilates for seniors is improved quality of life. By improving core strength, flexibility, balance, stability, joint pain, posture, stress, and energy, Pilates can help seniors to maintain their independence and improve their overall health and well-being.

Improved quality of life can mean different things for different seniors. For some, it may mean being able to participate in social activities or travel. For others, it may mean being able to perform everyday tasks, such as cooking or gardening, without pain or discomfort. Whatever the definition, Pilates can help seniors to achieve a higher quality of life.

Improved Brain Function

Research has shown that physical exercise can help to improve brain function, particularly in older adults. Pilates is no exception, and studies have shown that regular Pilates practice can lead to improved cognitive function and memory.

Pilates exercises that involve coordination and concentration can help to improve brain function and cognitive abilities. This can be particularly important for seniors who may be at risk for cognitive decline or dementia.

Reduced Risk of Chronic Diseases

Regular exercise, such as Pilates, can help to reduce the risk of chronic diseases, such as heart disease, diabetes, and osteoporosis. This is particularly important for seniors, who may be at a higher risk for these conditions.

Pilates exercises that focus on cardiovascular activity and muscle strengthening can help to reduce the risk of chronic diseases. In addition, the stress-reducing benefits of Pilates can help to reduce the risk of conditions related to stress, such as high blood pressure and anxiety.

How to get started with Pilates

If you're new to Pilates, it can be intimidating to get started, but with the right guidance, it can be a simple and enjoyable experience. This sub-chapter will provide some pointers on how to get started with Pilates.

Select a Qualified Instructor

Finding a qualified instructor is one of the most important steps in getting started with Pilates. A good instructor will be able to give you personalized attention, ensure that you are using proper form, and assist you in making safe progress.

When looking for a Pilates instructor, look for someone who is certified and has experience working with beginners. You can get recommendations from friends and family members, or you can search online for Pilates studios in your area.

Put on comfortable clothes.

It is critical to wear comfortable clothing that allows you to move freely when beginning Pilates. Avoid clothing that is too tight or restrictive, and instead choose breathable fabrics that wick sweat away.

You should also wear shoes or socks that are comfortable and allow you to move freely. Pilates is typically performed barefoot, so bring socks if you prefer to wear them.

Begin slowly.

If you are new to Pilates, it is important to begin slowly and gradually progress to more difficult exercises. Your instructor can assist you in creating a personalized workout plan that takes your fitness level and goals into account.

You may feel a little sore or fatigued after each session at first. This is normal and indicates that your body is adjusting to the new activity. However, if you experience pain or discomfort during or after a session, speak with your instructor and make any necessary adjustments to your routine.

Concentrate on Your Breathing

One of the fundamental principles of Pilates is to concentrate on your breathing. Proper breathing technique can help to improve your overall performance by improving the mind-body connection.

You should focus on breathing deeply and fully during Pilates exercises, inhaling through your nose and exhaling through your mouth. Your instructor can assist you in learning proper breathing techniques and ensuring that you breathe properly during each exercise.

Pay Attention to Your Body

As you begin your Pilates practice, pay attention to your body and adjust as needed. If you experience pain or discomfort while performing an exercise, stop and consult with your instructor.

Modifications or adjustments may be required in some cases to ensure that you are performing the exercises safely and effectively. Your instructor can assist you in modifying exercises and advising you on how to plan based on your specific needs.

Include Pilates in Your Routine

Pilates should be incorporated into your routine on a regular basis to reap the full benefits. This could imply going to classes several times a week or doing Pilates at home.

Have a good time!

Finally, remember to have fun with your Pilates practice. Pilates is an enjoyable and challenging form of exercise that can benefit your overall health and well-being.

You can get the most out of your Pilates practice and reap its many benefits by focusing on proper form, breathing, and listening to your bod

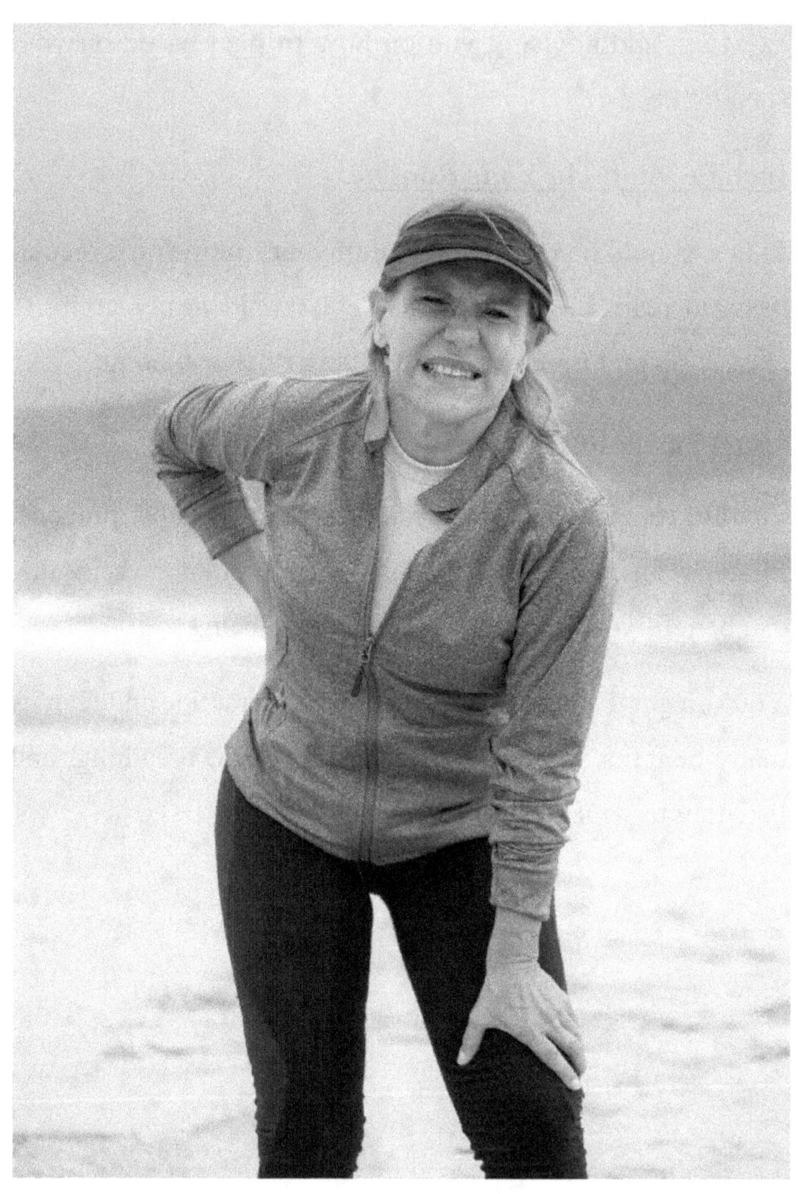

CHAPTER 2:

Essential Principles of Pilates

Joseph Pilates invented Pilates as a form of exercise in the early twentieth century. The system is intended to help people improve their strength, flexibility, balance, and posture. Pilates has grown in popularity around the world, and at the heart of the Pilates system are a number of fundamental principles that guide the practice and help to ensure maximum effectiveness and safety. In this chapter, we will delve deeper into these fundamental Pilates principles.

Concentration

Concentration is the first essential Pilates principle. Pilates exercises necessitate a great deal of mental focus and concentration. The goal is to concentrate on each movement while maintaining proper form and breathing. You can achieve better results and avoid injuries by remaining focused.

Pilates exercises are intended to be performed slowly and deliberately, with an emphasis on movement quality rather than quantity. This requires intense concentration because it is critical to be aware of each movement and its effects on the body.

Concentration is also essential for developing the mind-body connection, which is at the heart of the Pilates method. You can develop a greater awareness of your body and its capabilities by focusing on its movements and sensations.

Control

The second essential Pilates principle is control. Pilates exercises are slow and controlled, with an emphasis on quality of movement over quantity. The goal is to keep control of the movements while using the appropriate muscles and avoiding unnecessary tension.

Control is required to ensure that the exercises are done correctly and safely. You can avoid using the wrong muscles or creating unnecessary tension by focusing on the muscles that are being used.

Control is also essential for building strength and endurance. Exercises performed slowly and with control can help you build strength and endurance more effectively than exercises performed quickly or without proper form.

<u>Centering</u>

The third essential Pilates principle is centering. This principle states that all movements should begin in the center of the body, or the core. The abdominal muscles, lower back, hips, and buttocks are all part of the core. You can improve balance and stability, as well as overall body alignment, by focusing on the center of the body.

Maintaining proper form during Pilates exercises requires centering. By focusing on the core, you can ensure that each movement is initiated from the core, which aids in proper alignment and reduces the risk of injury.

Centering is also essential for developing core strength, which is required for good posture and balance. You can improve overall body function by focusing on the core muscles and developing greater strength and endurance in these muscles.

Breath

The fourth essential Pilates principle is breath. Breathing is an essential component of Pilates exercises because it improves oxygen flow, reduces tension, and increases mental focus. Pilates breathing entails breathing in through the nose and out through the mouth, with an emphasis on deep, controlled breaths.

During Pilates exercises, breathing is critical for maintaining focus and reducing tension. You can reduce stress and anxiety while also improving mental clarity and focus by breathing deeply and controlling your breath.

Breathing is also important for overall body function. You can increase energy levels and reduce fatigue by improving oxygen flow to the body. Deep breathing also promotes relaxation and improves circulation.

Precision

Precision is the fifth essential Pilates principle. Pilates exercises are precise and controlled, with an emphasis on proper alignment and form. Each movement should be executed precisely, using the appropriate muscles and avoiding unnecessary tension or strain.

Precision is required to ensure that the exercises are done correctly and safely. You can reduce the risk of injury and increase the effectiveness of the exercises by focusing on proper alignment and form.

Precision is also necessary for the development of body awareness. You can develop a greater awareness of your body and its capabilities by focusing on its movements and sensations. This can aid in the identification of areas of weakness or tension and the development of greater control and strength in those areas.

Flow

Flow is the sixth essential Pilates principle. Pilates exercises are intended to be performed in a continuous, flowing fashion, with an emphasis on smooth transitions between movements. This improves overall body coordination and movement fluidity.

Flow is essential for staying relaxed and at ease during Pilates exercises. You can reduce tension and stress while improving mental focus and clarity by maintaining a smooth and continuous flow of movement.

Flow is also essential for the development of overall body function. You can improve balance and stability while lowering your risk of falls and injuries by improving overall coordination and fluidity of movement.

Pilates' essential principles are critical to the Pilates system's effectiveness and safety. Concentration, control, breath, precision, and flow all contribute to a holistic approach to exercise that benefits people of all ages and fitness levels, but especially seniors.

Seniors can develop greater strength, flexibility, balance, and coordination, as well as improve overall body function, by adhering to these fundamental principles. Pilates is a low-impact form of exercise that is easy on the joints and appropriate for people of all physical abilities.

Fundamental Aspect of Pilates

Breathing techniques

Breathing is a fundamental aspect of Pilates that is frequently overlooked but is critical for reaping the full benefits of the exercises. Correct breathing during Pilates exercises can help seniors improve their overall health and fitness while also reducing stress and tension in the body. In this sub chapter, we will look at the importance of breathing in Pilates and offer some tips and techniques for seniors over 60 who want to improve their breathing while doing Pilates exercises.

What is the significance of breathing in Pilates?

Breathing is an important aspect of Pilates and is often referred to as the Pilates system's foundation. Proper breathing techniques aid in both providing the body with the oxygen it requires to fuel the muscles during exercise and removing waste products from the body.

Breathing also aids in relaxation and focus during exercise. We send a signal to the body to relax and release tension when we breathe deeply and rhythmically, which can help to reduce stress and improve mental focus.

Furthermore, correct breathing techniques can assist seniors in improving their posture, alignment, and core strength. We engage the diaphragm and other core muscles when we breathe deeply and fully, which can help to improve overall body stability and control.

Pilates breathing techniques

Breathing through the diaphragm

Diaphragmatic breathing, also known as belly breathing, is a breathing technique in which you breathe deeply into your abdomen rather than shallowly into your chest. This type of breathing encourages the diaphragm and other core muscles to contract, which can improve overall posture and alignment.

Sit or lie down in a comfortable position with one hand on your chest and the other on your belly to practice diaphragmatic breathing. Inhale deeply through your nose, feeling your belly expand and rise as you do so. Exhale slowly through your mouth, letting your belly drop as you do so. Repeat several times, paying attention to the sensation of the breath moving in and out of the body.

Ribcage respiration

Ribcage breathing is a technique that involves expanding the ribcage rather than just the belly as you inhale. This type of breathing can aid in the improvement of overall lung capacity as well as the release of tension in the upper back and shoulders.

Sit or stand with your arms at your sides to practice ribcage breathing. Inhale deeply through your nose, feeling your ribcage expand and lift as you do so. Exhale slowly through your mouth, allowing your ribcage to release and lower as you do so. Repeat several times, paying attention to the sensation of the breath moving in and out of the body.

Full-body respiration

Full-body breathing is a technique in which you breathe into your entire body, from your belly to your chest to your upper back and shoulders. This type of breathing can aid in the improvement of overall body awareness and the release of tension throughout the body.

Sit or stand with your arms at your sides to practice full-body breathing. Deeply inhale through the nose, allowing the breath to move into the belly, ribcage, upper back, and shoulders. Exhale slowly through your mouth, feeling the breath leave your upper back and shoulders, then your ribcage, and finally your belly. Repeat several times, focusing on the sensation of the breath moving throughout the body.

Taking deep breaths

Counting breaths is a technique that involves counting the length of each inhalation and exhalation and gradually increasing the length of the breaths over time. This type of breathing can aid in the improvement of overall lung capacity as well as the reduction of stress and tension in the body.

Sit or stand with your arms at your sides to practice counting breaths. Inhale deeply through the nose for four counts, then exhale slowly through the mouth for four counts. Repeat several times, paying attention to the sensation of the breath moving in and out of the body. As you become more comfortable with the technique, gradually lengthen the inhale and exhale to a count of six or eight.

Tips for Better Breathing During Pilates

Body relaxation

Take a moment before beginning any Pilates exercise to relax the body and release any tension or stress. Close your eyes, take several deep breaths, and concentrate on the sensation of the breath moving in and out of your body. This can help the body prepare for exercise and improve breathing efficiency.

Keep your spine in a neutral position.

Maintaining a neutral spine, with the natural curves of the spine in proper alignment, can aid in improving breathing efficiency and reducing body tension. Throughout each exercise, keep your core muscles engaged and your pelvis stable.

Breathing and movement should be coordinated.

Breathing is frequently coordinated with movement in Pilates, with the inhale occurring during the preparation phase and the exhale occurring during the exertion phase. Focus on the rhythm and timing of the breath, and try to coordinate the breath as much as possible with the movement.

Try not to hold your breath.

Holding your breath during exercise can cause muscle tension and discomfort, as well as reduce the effectiveness of the exercise. Maintain a rhythmic breathing pattern throughout each exercise, and avoid holding your breath or breathing too shallowly.

Proper Alignment and Posture

Our bodies may become more susceptible to aches, pains, and stiffness as we age, and proper alignment and posture can help to reduce discomfort and improve overall health and fitness. Poor posture and alignment can cause a variety of physical issues, including back pain, neck pain, shoulder pain, and joint pain. Furthermore, poor alignment and posture can impair balance and stability, increasing the risk of falls and injury.

Proper alignment and posture are especially important for seniors over the age of 60 because aging can cause changes in the structure and function of the body. These changes may include decreased bone density, muscle mass, flexibility, and range of motion. Seniors can improve their overall health and fitness, reduce discomfort, and lower their risk of injury by maintaining proper alignment and posture during Pilates exercises.

Guidelines for achieving and maintaining proper posture and alignment during Pilates exercises

Engage the abdominal muscles.

Pilate's proper alignment and posture begin with the core muscles, which include the abdominal, back, and pelvic floor muscles. Engaging these muscles can aid in pelvic and spine stabilization, posture improvement, and injury prevention. Draw the navel toward the spine and lift the pelvic floor muscles to engage the core muscles.

Keep your spine in a neutral position.

Maintaining a neutral spine with the natural curves of the spine in proper alignment can help to reduce back, neck, and shoulder tension and discomfort. Maintain a neutral spine by keeping your shoulders relaxed, chest lifted, and lower back supported.

Adjust the hips and pelvis.

Proper hip and pelvic alignment are critical for overall balance, stability, and posture. Engage the core muscles and keep the hips level and squared to the front to align the hips and pelvis.

Assemble the shoulders and arms.

Proper shoulder and arm alignment can help to reduce tension and discomfort in the neck and shoulders, as well as improve overall posture. Keep the shoulders relaxed and down, and the arms in line with the shoulders, to align the shoulders and arms.

Maintain proper head and neck alignment

Proper head and neck alignment are critical for reducing tension and discomfort in the neck and shoulders, as well as improving overall posture. Keep the chin level and the head aligned with the spine to maintain proper head and neck alignment.

Concentrate on proper breathing technique.

Maintaining proper alignment and posture during Pilates exercises requires proper breathing technique. Seniors can improve their overall health and fitness, reduce tension and discomfort, and improve posture and alignment by focusing on the rhythm and timing of their breath.

Core Engagement and Stability

The core muscles, which include the muscles of the abdomen, back, and pelvic floor, are essential for proper alignment and posture, as well as for overall movement and mobility. By engaging the core muscles during Pilates exercises, seniors can improve their overall health and fitness, reduce discomfort, and reduce the risk of injury.

Tips for achieving and maintaining proper core engagement and stability during Pilates exercises

Focus on the breath

Proper breathing technique is essential for achieving and maintaining proper core engagement and stability during Pilates exercises. By focusing on the rhythm and timing of the breath, seniors can engage the core muscles and improve overall stability and balance.

Engage the pelvic floor muscles

Engaging the pelvic floor muscles is essential for proper core engagement and stability, particularly for seniors over 60. By lifting and contracting the pelvic floor muscles, seniors can improve overall stability and balance, as well as reduce the risk of incontinence.

Engage the abdominal muscles

Engaging the abdominal muscles is essential for proper core engagement and stability during Pilates exercises. By drawing the navel toward the spine and lifting the lower abdominal muscles, seniors can engage the core muscles and improve overall stability and balance.

Engage the back muscles

Engaging the back muscles is also essential for proper core engagement and stability during Pilates exercises. By lifting and lengthening the spine and engaging the muscles of the upper and lower back, seniors can improve overall stability and balance.

Maintain proper alignment and posture

Proper alignment and posture are essential for achieving and maintaining proper core engagement and stability during Pilates exercises. By maintaining a neutral spine and aligning the hips, shoulders, and head, seniors can engage the core muscles and improve overall stability and balance.

Use props and modifications

Props and modifications can also be used to achieve and maintain proper core engagement and stability during Pilates exercises. For example, using a Pilates ball or foam roller can help to engage the core muscles and improve overall stability and balance. Additionally, modifications can be used to make exercises more accessible and to reduce the risk of injury.

Mind-Body Connection

The ability to focus on the present moment and connect with one's body can help to reduce stress and anxiety, improve mental clarity, and improve overall health and well-being. Our bodies may become more prone to aches, pains, and stiffness as we age, and the mind-body connection can help to alleviate discomfort and improve overall health and fitness.

Furthermore, the mind-body connection can improve balance and stability, lowering the risk of falls and injury. Seniors can improve their overall health and fitness, reduce discomfort, and lower their risk of injury by connecting the mind and body during Pilates exercises.

Tips for establishing and maintaining a strong mind-body connection while performing Pilates exercises

Concentrate on your breathing.

During Pilates exercises, proper breathing technique is critical for achieving and maintaining a strong mind-body connection. Seniors can connect with their bodies and improve mental clarity and focus by focusing on the rhythm and timing of their breath.

Exercise mindfulness.

The practice of focusing on the present moment and being aware of one's thoughts and feelings is known as mindfulness. Seniors can connect with their bodies and reduce stress and anxiety by practicing mindfulness during Pilates exercises.

Consider the movement.

The practice of imagining a movement before performing it is known as visualization. Seniors can connect with their bodies and improve overall movement and mobility by visualizing the movement during Pilates exercises.

Make use of positive affirmations.

Affirmations that promote positive thoughts and feelings are known as positive affirmations. Seniors can connect with their bodies and improve their mental clarity and focus by using positive affirmations during Pilates exercises.

Pay attention to your body.

Listening to the body during Pilates exercises is critical for achieving and maintaining a strong mind-body connection. Seniors can connect with their bodies and reduce discomfort by paying attention to their bodies and responding to their needs.

Use your senses.

Using the senses, such as sight, sound, and touch, during Pilates exercises can also help to strengthen the mind-body connection. Seniors, for example, can concentrate on the sound of their breath or the sensation of their muscles contracting and relaxing.

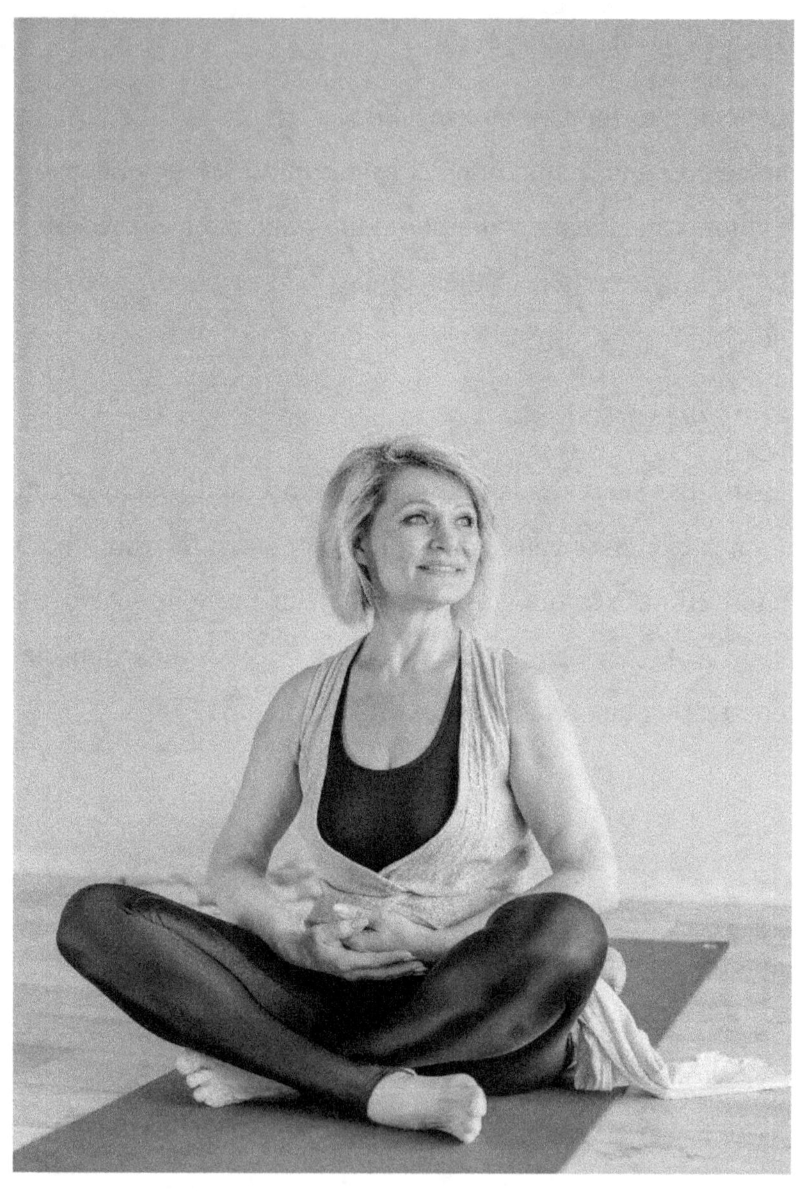

CHAPTER 3:

Pilates Exercises for Seniors

Pilates is a gentle yet effective way for seniors to stay active, improve their posture, and lower their risk of injury and falls. This chapter will look at some Pilates exercises that are great for seniors.

The One Hundred

The Hundred is a classic Pilates exercise that is great for warming up the body and strengthening the core. Begin by lying on your back with your knees bent, your feet flat on the floor, and your arms by your sides. Extend your arms straight out in front of you, lifting your head and shoulders off the ground. Begin pumping your arms up and down for five counts, then out for five counts. Rep for a total of 100 times.

The Hundred is a difficult exercise that strengthens the core, arms, and cardiovascular system. It is ideal for seniors who want to increase their energy and stamina while improving their overall fitness level.

Roll-Up

The Roll-Up is an excellent exercise for developing core strength, increasing spine flexibility, and stretching the hamstrings. Begin by lying on your back and extending your legs straight out in front of you. Raise your arms to the ceiling and slowly roll your spine up and away from the ground, reaching your arms towards your toes. Hold this position for a few seconds before slowly rolling back down to the starting position.

The Roll-Up is a difficult exercise that requires core muscle control and stability. It is ideal for seniors who want to improve their posture, alleviate back pain, and gain flexibility.

Single Leg Circle

The Single Leg Circle exercise is great for increasing hip and leg strength and flexibility. Begin by lying on your back with your arms at your sides and your legs straight up in the air to perform this exercise. Circulate your right leg clockwise, keeping your left leg straight and still. Repeat for 5-10 circles before switching to the other leg.

The Single Leg Circle is a gentle yet effective exercise that works the hip and leg muscles while also improving lower body flexibility. It is ideal for seniors who want to maintain hip and leg mobility while reducing the risk of falls and injury.

The Spine Stretch

The Spine Stretch is an excellent exercise for improving posture and spine flexibility. Begin by sitting on the ground with your legs straight out in front of you to perform this exercise. Inhale deeply and raise your arms to the ceiling. Exhale and extend your arms forward, stretching your spine and reaching for your toes. Hold this position for a few seconds before slowly rolling back up to the starting position.

The Spine Stretch is a gentle exercise that helps to relax the back and neck muscles, improves posture, and increases spine flexibility. It is ideal for seniors who want to keep their spine mobile and reduce their risk of back pain and injury.

The Shoulder Bridge

The Shoulder Bridge is an excellent exercise for increasing core strength and spine and hip flexibility. Begin by lying on your back with your knees bent and your feet flat on the floor to perform this exercise. Raise your hips to the ceiling while keeping your arms at your sides. Hold this position for a few seconds before slowly rolling back down to the starting position.

The Shoulder Bridge is a difficult exercise that strengthens the core, glutes, and hip muscles while also improving stability and balance. It is ideal for seniors who want to maintain hip and spine mobility while reducing the risk of falls and injury.

Side-Lying Leg Lifts

Side-Lying Leg Lifts are an excellent exercise for strengthening and toning the hip and leg muscles, which are important for maintaining mobility and stability in later life. Begin this exercise by lying on your side with your bottom arm straight out and your head resting on it. Lift your top leg to the ceiling while keeping your foot flexed, then lower it back down. Repeat for 10-15 before switching.

Side-Lying Leg Lifts are a low-impact exercise that strengthens the hip and leg muscles while also improving balance and stability. It is ideal for seniors who want to maintain lower-body mobility while reducing the risk of falls and injury.

Swan

The Swan is an excellent exercise for increasing upper body strength, posture, and spine flexibility. Begin by lying on your stomach with your hands under your shoulders to perform this exercise. Lift your chest off the ground while keeping your arms straight. Exhale and return to the starting position.

The Swan is a difficult exercise that requires core muscle control and stability, as well as upper body strength. It is ideal for seniors who want to improve their posture, reduce back pain, and strengthen and stretch their upper body.

The Seated Spinal Twist

The Seated Spinal Twist is a great exercise for improving spine mobility, promoting good digestion and detoxification, and reducing stress and tension. Begin by sitting on the ground with your legs straight out in front of you to perform this exercise. Place your foot on the outside of your left knee and bend your right knee. Inhale and raise your left arm to the ceiling, then exhale and twist your body towards your right knee, supporting yourself with your right hand. Hold this position for a moment before switching to the opposite side.

The Seated Spinal Twist is a gentle exercise that promotes good digestion and detoxification while also reducing stress and tension. It is ideal for seniors who want to keep their spine mobile and reduce their risk of back pain and injury.

Warm-Up Exercises

Any exercise program, including Pilates, must start with a warm-up. They increase the effectiveness of the workout, lower the risk of injury, and prepare the body for more strenuous exercise. Pilates warm-up exercises are crucial for seniors because they may have limited flexibility or mobility. The warm-up exercises listed below are perfect for seniors to perform before beginning their Pilates workout.

Shoulder Rolls

Shoulder rolls are a great warm-up exercise that enhances shoulder and upper back mobility. Start by assuming a shoulder-width distance between your feet and keeping your arms at your sides. Lifting your shoulders toward your ears while inhaling, roll them back and down while exhaling. After performing this motion 10 to 15 times, change the direction.

Arm Circles

Arm circles are a quick but effective warm-up exercise that promotes better shoulder and arm mobility. Start by assuming a shoulder-width distance between your feet and keeping your arms at your sides. Exhale as you circle your arms forward after inhaling and raising them to shoulder height. After performing this motion 10 to 15 times, change the direction.

The Cat-Cow Stretch

The Cat-Cow stretch is a great pre-exercise that increases the spine's flexibility and mobility. Begin by getting down on all fours, placing your knees beneath your hips and your hands under your shoulders. Inhale, arch your back, and point your tailbone and chest upward. Bring your head toward your knees as you exhale and round your spine. 10-15 times should be spent repeating this motion.

Hip circles

Hip circles are a fantastic warm-up exercise that enhances lower back and hip mobility. Put your hands on your hips and begin by standing with your feet shoulder-width apart. Circulate your hips to the right as you inhale, then to the left as you exhale. After performing this motion 10 to 15 times, change the direction.

Rolled Ankles

An easy warm-up exercise that helps to increase ankle and foot mobility is the rolling of the ankles. Starting off, place your hands on your hips and stand with your feet hip-width apart. Lifting your left foot off the ground while inhaling will cause your ankle to circle to the right. Circulate your left ankle as you exhale. Repeat this motion for 10-15 repetitions, and then switch to the other foot.

Knee Lift

Knee lifts are a great warm-up exercise that helps to increase hip and knee mobility. Starting off, place your hands on your hips and stand with your feet hip-width apart. Inhale, bringing your right knee up to your chest; exhale, bringing it back down. 15 to 20 repetitions of this motion should be performed before switching to the other knee.

Pelvic Tilt

The pelvic tilt is a great exercise for senior citizens because it enhances stability and core strength. Laying on your back with your knees bent and your feet flat on the ground is a good place to start. Tilt your pelvis toward your ribs while inhaling, then toward your feet while exhaling. 10-15 times should be spent repeating this motion.

Leg circles

Leg circles are a low-impact exercise that strengthens the core and increases hip mobility. To begin, lie on your back with your legs straight up towards the ceiling and your arms at your sides. Inhale and circle your right leg to the right, down and around, and back up. Exhale and repeat the motion to the left. After performing this movement 10 to 15 times, switch to the other leg.

The single-leg bridge

The single-leg bridge is a great exercise for senior citizens because it boosts stability and core strength. Laying on your back with your knees bent and your feet flat on the ground is a good place to start. Lift your left foot off the ground while inhaling, then exhale while lifting your hips upwards. Exhale after bringing your hips back down, then inhale after moving your right foot in the same way. 10-15 times should be spent repeating this motion.

Arm Reaches

Arm reaches are a low-impact exercise that strengthens the core and increases shoulder mobility. Start by assuming a chair-seated position with your hands on your hips and your feet flat on the floor. Your right arm should be raised toward the ceiling as you inhale; it should be lowered back down as you exhale. Repeat this motion with your left arm. 10-15 times should be spent repeating this motion.

Spine Twist

The spine twist is a great exercise for senior citizens because it helps to strengthen the core and improve spinal mobility. Start by assuming a chair-seated position with your hands on your hips and your feet flat on the floor. Twist your torso to the right as you inhale, then to the left as you exhale. 10-15 times should be spent repeating this motion.

Knee Folds

Knee folds are a low-impact exercise that strengthens the core and increases hip mobility. Laying on your back with your knees bent and your feet flat on the ground is a good place to start. Lift your feet off the ground while inhaling, and then exhale while bringing your knees up to your chest.

Take a breath, bring your feet back down, then exhale and repeat. 10-15 times should be spent repeating this motion.

Standing exercises

Seniors can incorporate Pilates into their daily routine by performing standing exercises. These exercises are especially beneficial because they help seniors improve their balance, stability, and posture, which can help them maintain their independence and avoid falls. The following are some senior-friendly Pilates standing exercises.

Arm Reach from a Standing Position

Standing arm reaches are an excellent exercise for seniors because they help to improve shoulder mobility and core strength. Begin by standing hip-width apart with your arms at your sides. Inhale and raise your right arm to the ceiling, then exhale and lower it again. Repeat this movement with your left arm. Repeat this motion for about 10-15 times.

Standing Leg Raises

Standing leg raises are a low-impact exercise that helps to improve hip mobility and core strength. Start by placing your hands on your hips and standing with your feet hip-width apart. Inhale and extend your right leg out to the side, then exhale and return it to the starting position. Repeat this movement with your left leg. Repeat this motion for about 10-15 times.

The Standing Hamstring Curl.

The standing hamstring curl is an excellent exercise for seniors that helps to improve hip mobility and core strength. Begin by placing your hands on your hips and standing with your feet hip-width apart. Inhale and raise your right heel to your buttocks, then exhale and lower it back down. Repeat this movement with your left heel. Repeat this motion for about 10-15 times.

Standing Lunge

The standing lunge is an excellent exercise for seniors that helps to improve leg and hip strength and stability. Begin by placing your hands on your hips and standing with your feet hip-width apart. Inhale and take a step forward with your right foot, then exhale and bend your right knee, lowering your body to the ground. Inhale and return your right foot to the starting position, then exhale and repeat with your left foot. Repeat this motion for about 10-15 times.

Standing Side Stretches

Standing side stretches are an excellent exercise for seniors because they help to improve spine mobility and core strength. Begin by standing hip-width apart with your arms at your sides. Inhale and raise your right arm to the ceiling, then exhale and bend to the left, reaching your left hand down to the ground. Return to the starting position by inhaling, then exhaling and repeating the motion to the right. Repeat this motion for about 10-15 times.

Mat Exercises

For seniors over 60, Mat Exercises are an essential part of their Pilates routine. They provide a gentle yet efficient method to develop the core, enhance balance, increase flexibility, and improve mobility in general. Seniors can benefit from the following mat exercises:

Single-Leg Circles: This exercise is excellent for strengthening the core and enhancing hip mobility. Lie on your back with your legs straight up in the air and your arms at your sides. Five times in a clockwise direction, then five times in a counterclockwise direction, circle your left leg. Repeat while changing legs.

Roll Like a Ball: This exercise is excellent for enhancing control and balance. Kneel down on your mat with your feet flat on the surface. Lifting your feet off the mat requires you to hold onto your shins and round your spine. Reposition yourself seated by rolling back onto your shoulders. It should be repeated ten times.

Spine Stretch: This exercise is excellent for enhancing spinal mobility and posture. Sit on your mat with your arms reaching down to your feet and your legs straight out in front of you. Exhale while rounding your spine and extending your hands toward your toes. Inhale and lengthen your spine. Ten times should be repeated.

Swimming is a great exercise for building back strength and enhancing mobility in general. Stretch your arms and legs while lying on your stomach. Ten times, raise your arms and legs off the floor and flutter them up and down.

Teaser: This exercise is fantastic for developing core strength and balance. Lay on your back with your legs straight out in front of you and your arms raised above your head. Roll back down to the starting position after rolling up to a seated position and balancing on your sit bones. Repeat 10 times.

The side plank is a fantastic exercise for oblique muscle development and balance enhancement. Lay on your side with your legs stacked on top of one another and your elbow directly under your shoulder. For ten seconds, raise your hips off the floor. Then switch sides once more.

Leg Pull: This exercise is excellent for improving hip mobility and strengthening the core. Start in a plank position with your feet straight behind you and your hands directly beneath your shoulders. Maintaining straight legs, raise your hips toward the ceiling for 10 seconds. Ten repetitions should be performed before lowering back to the starting position.

Roll-Ups: This exercise is excellent for strengthening the core and enhancing spinal mobility. Lay on your back with your legs straight out in front of you and your arms raised above your head. Roll up until you are seated, then roll back down to where you were when you first started. Ten times should be repeated.

Modifications for Different Levels of Fitness

<u>Beginner Modifications</u>: It's crucial to start with the fundamentals and perform exercises more slowly for seniors who are new to Pilates. Among the modifications are:

Use props: You can support your body while exercising by using props like cushions or pillows. For support during core exercises, one can place a pillow under the head and neck, for instance.

Reduce range of motion: Until they feel more at ease with the movement, seniors can perform exercises with a reduced range of motion.

Exercises for seniors who are just starting out can be made easier by using less resistance, such as lighter weights or resistance bands.

Intermediate Modifications: Seniors who are looking for a challenge and have Pilates experience can modify exercises to make them harder. Among the modifications are:

Heavier Weights: Seniors can use heavier weights or increase the resistance on resistance bands to make exercises more difficult.

Lengthen range of motion: To work their muscles harder and become more flexible, seniors can engage in exercises with a wider range of motion.

Add complexity: Seniors can make exercises more challenging by including movements like twisting or reaching.

Advanced Pilates: Seniors with advanced Pilates experience and high levels of fitness can modify exercises to make them more difficult. Among the modifications are:

Include balance: To test balance and stability, exercises can be done on one leg or with one arm.

Increased intensity can be achieved by seniors performing their exercises more quickly or for a longer period of time.

<u>Use unstable surfaces</u>: To test balance and core strength, seniors can perform exercises on unstable surfaces like a stability ball.

All seniors should seek advice from a trained Pilates instructor before beginning any exercise program, particularly if they have any health issues or physical restrictions. Exercises can be altered by a trainer to meet individual needs and ensure correct form and technique.

Other adjustments can be made to accommodate various physical conditions in addition to those that are already mentioned. For instance:

Arthritis: Seniors who suffer from arthritis can adapt their workouts by using a softer surface, tower cushion for extra support.

Osteoporosis: Seniors with osteoporosis should modify their workouts by staying away from twists and forward bends that put too much strain on the spine.

Joint pain: Exercises can be modified for seniors with joint pain by going more slowly or using less resistance.

CHAPTER 4

Warm-Up Exercises

Neck Rolls

Neck rolls can be incorporated into any Pilates program for seniors over 60 as a quick but effective warm-up exercise. This easy exercise improves range of motion and warms up the neck muscles, lowering the risk of injury during more challenging Pilates exercises. We'll go over the advantages of neck rolls, how to do them properly, and a few variations for people of various fitness levels in this chapter.

Neck Rolls Benefits

Our muscles and joints stiffen as we age, and we lose mobility and flexibility. Neck rolls encourage better posture and lower the risk of pain or injury by releasing tension and stiffness in the neck, shoulders, and upper back.

The following are some rewards of neck rolls:

Reduces tension in the Shoulders and Neck

Neck rolls help to release tension and stiffness in the neck and shoulder muscles and improve blood circulation. Senior citizens who spend a lot of time sitting or have limited mobility may find this to be especially beneficial.

Expands your Range of Motion

Our neck muscles tend to weaken with age, limiting our range of motion. Increased range of motion from neck rolls can make it easier for seniors to perform daily tasks.

Encourages Good Posture

Neck rolls aid in extending the neck and enhancing posture. Chronic pain, headaches, and exhaustion can all be caused by poor posture. You can help to improve your posture and lower your risk of developing these problems by including neck rolls in your Pilates regimen.

Lowers the Possibility of Injury

Seniors can lower their risk of injury when performing more strenuous Pilates exercises by warming up their neck muscles and increasing their flexibility.

How to Roll Your Neck

These easy steps will show you how to do neck rolls:

-Put your arms by your sides, sit up straight, and relax your shoulders.

-Bring your chin down to your chest gradually and hold for a few seconds.

-Roll your head slowly to the right, bringing your right ear toward your right shoulder while maintaining a relaxed posture.

-Hold for a short while, then tilt your head back and look up at the ceiling.

-Bring your left ear toward your left shoulder as you slowly turn your head to the left.

-Lower your chin toward your chest and bring your head back down.

-Roll your head in the opposite direction, repeat the exercise.

Guidelines for Proper Form

Maintaining proper form throughout the exercise is crucial for performing neck rolls safely and effectively. For proper form, consider the following advice:

Continue to relax your shoulders.

Make sure to maintain a relaxed posture throughout the exercise and to avoid hunching or tensing your shoulders.

Move Gently and Gradually

Slowly and gently rolling your neck is the best way to relieve tension in your neck muscles. A jerky motion or a rapid head roll should be avoided to prevent injury.

Avoid Overextending

Rolling your head back or to the side should be done gently. Do not overstretch your neck muscles as this could result in pain or damage.

Inhale Deeply

Throughout the exercise, be sure to take deep breaths, slowly inhaling and exhaling as you roll your head.

Adaptations for Various Fitness Levels

Various fitness levels can use modified neck rolls. Here are a few changes:

Seniors who find it difficult to stand up or who have limited mobility can perform neck rolls while seated. Simply take a seat in a chair with your feet flat on the floor and repeat the previous steps.

Shoulder shrugs can be a good substitute for seniors who find it difficult to perform neck rolls. Simply bring your shoulders up to your ears, hold for a short period of time, and roll repeatedly.

Guidelines for safely performing neck rolls

Neck rolls are a gentle, helpful warm-up exercise, but it's important to perform them safely to prevent harm. Here are some pointers for safely performing neck rolls:

-Beginning with small movements will allow you to gradually increase the range of motion as your neck muscles warm up. If you're new to neck rolls, start with small movements.

-Avoid jerky movements when performing neck rolls; they should always be gentle. Don't try to force your head into an uncomfortable position or strain your neck beyond its normal range of motion.

-Maintain a relaxed posture: When practicing Neck Rolls, be sure to maintain a relaxed posture with your shoulders, not hunched up around your ears. This will lessen the likelihood of shoulder and neck tension developing.

-Breathe deeply: When performing Neck Rolls, as with any Pilates exercise, it's crucial to breathe deeply and rhythmically. Roll your head back towards your chest while taking a slow, deep breath through your nose and lifting your chin to the ceiling.

-If necessary, adjust the exercise: It's important to adjust Neck Rolls to meet your needs if you have any shoulder or neck injuries or conditions. Consult your Pilates instructor or a medical professional for advice on how to safely modify the exercise.

A quick and efficient warm-up exercise for seniors, neck rolls helps to increase their range of motion, release tension, and improve blood flow to their head and neck. Seniors can improve their overall flexibility, strength, and posture by regularly performing Neck Rolls as part of a Pilates routine, which can help to lower the risk of falls, injuries, and other age-related health issues. Always practice neck rolls safely and conscientiously, beginning with small motions and progressively extending the range of motion over time. Neck rolls can be an effective tool for maintaining general health and well-being in seniors with regular practice and a mindful approach.

Shoulder Rolls

Exercises like the shoulder roll help to mobilize the shoulder joint and enhance blood flow in the upper body. Seniors who suffer from stiff shoulders or upper backs, as well as those who have poor posture, can benefit from this exercise. Seniors who spend a lot of time sitting or standing in the same position may find that the shoulder roll exercise is a good way to relieve stress and tension in their neck and shoulders.

To incorporate the shoulder roll exercise into your Pilates warm-up routine, follow these steps:

Step 1: To begin, place your feet shoulder-width apart while standing up straight. Place your arms loosely and at your sides.

Step 2: After taking a long, deep breath in, lift your shoulders up toward your ears.

Step 3: Remain in this position with your shoulders for a short while, feeling the stretch and tension in your upper back and neck.

Step 4: Roll your shoulders back while taking a breath in, squeezing your shoulder blades together.

Step 5: Keep rolling your shoulders back until they are in the position they were in at the beginning.

Step 6: Continue the exercise while exhaling, rolling your shoulders to the front and then back to the starting position.

Step 7: Carry out 5 to 10 repetitions of the shoulder roll exercise.

<u>Advice on Form and Technique</u>

Even though the shoulder roll exercise is straightforward, using the right form and technique will help you get the most out of the exercise and prevent injuries. Observe the following advice:

-Aim to move slowly and deliberately throughout the exercise. Do not jerk your shoulders or move too quickly. Concentrate on the stretch and tension in your upper back and neck as you move slowly and under control.

-Rolling your shoulders should only go as far as is comfortable for you. Avoid overextending your shoulders to avoid risking harm to yourself.

-Keep your neck relaxed: As you perform the exercise, try to keep your neck relaxed and refrain from tensing up. Keep working with your shoulders.

-Breathe deeply, lifting your shoulders toward your ears as you inhale and rolling them back and down as you exhale. You can unwind and let go of tension in your upper body by doing this.

Shoulder rolls: Their advantages

Reduces hunching or slouching: Shoulder rolls help to mobilize and loosen up the muscles in the upper back and neck, which can help improve posture.

Increases range of motion: The shoulder roll exercise aids in increasing the shoulder joint's range of motion, which can be especially beneficial for seniors who are experiencing stiffness or limited mobility.

Releases tension and stress: Shoulder rolls can be particularly helpful for seniors who are experiencing chronic pain or discomfort because they can help release tension and stress in the upper body.

Increases blood flow and circulation in the upper body: Shoulder rolls help to do this by moving the shoulder joint and upper back.

<u>Let's now discuss a few different shoulder roll exercise variations.</u>

Shoulder circles: Start by rotating your shoulders in a circle in the forward direction, then move on to the backward direction. Make 5–10 circular motions in each direction.

Squeeze your shoulder blades together while standing or sitting with your arms at your sides. Pull your shoulders back and down while squeezing your shoulder blades together. Hold for some time, then let go. 5–10 times, then stop.

Arm circles: Hold your arms at shoulder height straight out to the sides. Make a series of small, forward-rotating circles with your arms, then switch to backward-rotating circles. Make 5–10 circular motions in each direction.

Stretch your shoulders by placing your left hand on your right shoulder and your right hand on your left. Pull your elbows back and gently press your shoulders down and away from your ears. Hold for some time, then let go. 5–10 times, then stop.

When performing these exercises, keep in mind that it's crucial to pay attention to your body and move at your own pace. Stop the exercise and seek medical advice if you feel any pain or discomfort.

Arm Circles

A quick but effective warm-up exercise, arm circles can help get the upper body ready for more demanding activity. The exercise, which can be performed in a variety of positions, involves making circles with the arms as the name suggests. The exercise can improve circulation, encourage relaxation, and stretch and loosen up the shoulders, arms, and upper back.

You can stand with your feet hip-width apart and your arms outstretched at shoulder height to perform arm circles. Simply start making small circles with your arms from this point forward, enlarging the circles as you go. To target different muscles, you can change the movement's direction and repeat it several times. You can also experiment with holding your arms in different positions, like in front of your body or above your head.

Although arm circles are a low-impact exercise, if done incorrectly they can still cause some strain on the shoulders and upper back. It's crucial to keep your form correct throughout the exercise and to stop if you feel any pain or discomfort.

How to Safely Perform Arm Circles

There are a few crucial pointers and recommendations to remember when performing arm circles safely:

Start Slowly: As you warm up, it's best to start with small circles and gradually increase their size. This will aid in avoiding any discomfort or strain.

Focus on Form: It's crucial to maintain a relaxed neck and slightly bent elbows throughout the exercise. Instead of swinging or using momentum, you should be making the circles with your arm muscles.

Avoid Overstretching: It's important to warm up and stretch your upper body, but you shouldn't ever stretch yourself too far or until you feel pain. It's best to stop exercising and take a short break if you experience any strain or soreness.

Breathe Deeply: Pay close attention to your breathing throughout the motion. This may aid in body relaxation and improve circulation.

Stop if You Feel Lightheaded: When performing arm circles, some people, especially beginners, may feel lightheaded or dizzy. It is best to stop and take a break if you feel lightheaded or uncomfortable.

Benefits of Arm Circles for Seniors

After discussing safe arm circle techniques, let's examine the advantages arm circles can offer to people over 60:

Increased Range of Motion: Arm circles can aid in increasing the flexibility and range of motion in the upper back, shoulders, and arms. Seniors who might feel stiffness or discomfort in these areas can benefit most from this.

Circulation: Making arm circles can help to improve circulation and blood flow in the upper body. This may facilitate the muscles' and joints' healing by reducing inflammation.

Lower the Risk of Injury: Arm circles can help to lower the risk of injury by warming up the upper body prior to more strenuous exercise. Seniors, who may be more prone to injuries due to age-related changes in muscle strength and bone density, should pay particular attention to this.

Improved Posture: By working the shoulders and upper back muscles, arm circles can also help to improve posture. Seniors who may spend a lot of time sitting or hunched over, which can result in poor posture and related health issues, may find this to be especially helpful.

Promote Relaxation and raise mind-body Awareness: Last but not least, arm circles can be a fantastic way to promote relaxation and raise mind-body awareness. Seniors can reduce stress and anxiety by concentrating on their movements and taking deep breaths, which can have numerous advantages for their general health and wellbeing.

Adding Arm Circles to Your Pilates Exercises

There are a few things to consider if you're a senior over 60 who wants to include arm circles in your Pilates routine:

Start Slowly: As previously mentioned, it is best to begin with small circles and progressively increase the size as you warm up. This will aid in avoiding any discomfort or strain.

Focus on Form: Rather than relying on momentum or swinging, keep your form correct the entire time and make the circles with your muscles.

Change Your Position: You can change your position by holding your arms in front of you or above your head, or you can change the direction of the circles to work different muscles.

Spinal Twist

The spinal twist is a Pilates exercise that has you sit on the ground and twist your upper body from side to side. It focuses on the back, hip, and core muscles, which can help to ease back pain, increase spinal mobility, and encourage upright posture. Although the exercise is easy to do, it must be done properly to maximize the benefits and prevent injury.

Instructions for the Spinal Twist

The steps for the spinal twist are as follows:

-Your hands should be resting on your thighs as you sit on the floor with your legs out in front of you.

-Imagine that a string attached to the top of your head is lifting you upward as you take a deep breath and lengthen your spine.

-Exhale, then start to rotate your upper body to the right while starting with your abdominal muscles as the propulsion. Legs and hips should always be pointed forward.

-Put your left hand on your right thigh and your right hand on the ground behind you. If necessary, deepen the twist using your hands.

-Take a few long, deep breaths while holding the position, then exhale as you slowly return to the starting position.

-With your right hand on your left thigh and your left hand on the floor behind you, twist to the opposite side as you exhale. Go through the sequence, switching sides each time.

Guidelines for Safely Executing the Spinal Twist

Keep the following advice in mind to perform the spinal twist safely and effectively:

Warm up first: It's important to warm up the body with some gentle stretching or low-impact movements before performing the spinal twist or any other exercise. By doing this, you'll be able to avoid injuries and get your muscles ready for the next exercise.

Use your core muscles: Instead of relying on momentum or twisting too far, start the twist by using your abdominal muscles. By doing so, you'll protect your back and make sure the right muscles are being used.

Maintaining stability with your hips and legs will help you maintain your forward-facing posture as you twist. This will make it easier to target the back and core muscles.

If you need to, use a cushion or yoga block to support your hips or lower back if you have limited mobility or find it difficult to sit comfortably on the floor.

Breathe deeply: Pay attention to inhaling and exhaling fully as you perform the spinal twist. This will encourage relaxation and well-being and help to oxygenate the muscles.

Benefit of Spinal Twist for Seniors.

The spinal twist can provide a number of advantages, such as:

Improved spinal flexibility and mobility: The spinal twist can help the spine become more flexible and mobile, which is especially advantageous for seniors who might experience back pain or stiffness.

Reduced back pain: The spinal twist can aid in reducing back pain and enhancing posture by stretching and strengthening the back muscles.

Better Digestion: The spinal twist's twisting motion can aid in stimulating the digestive system, which can be especially advantageous for seniors who may have digestive issues.

Increased Circulation: The spinal twist's deep breathing and twisting motion can aid in boosting the blood flow to the muscles and oxygenating them, which can help to improve general health and wellbeing.

Balance: Balance and coordination can be strengthened over time by practicing the spinal twist, which calls for both of these abilities.

Reduced Stress and Tension: The spinal twist's deep breathing and stretching can help the body relax and feel better overall by reducing stress and tension.

Better Posture: The spinal twist can help to improve posture and lower the risk of falls or other accidents by stretching and strengthening the back muscles.

Leg Swings

Benefit of Leg Swings for Seniors

Improved Mobility: Leg swings can help increase hip joint range of motion and mobility, which is especially advantageous for seniors who have pain or stiffness there. Seniors can gently stretch and mobilize the hip joint by swinging the leg side to side and back and forth, which will lessen pain and increase flexibility.

Leg swings require balance and coordination, which can help to gradually improve these abilities over time. Seniors can lower their risk of falls and other injuries by performing this exercise frequently to increase their ability to maintain stability and control in the lower body.

Muscles that are strengthened: Leg swings can help to strengthen the muscles in the lower body, such as the glutes, quadriceps, and hip flexors. Seniors can improve their overall physical health and make other physical activities easier to perform by using these muscles during the exercise.

Increase Circulation in the lower body: Leg swings can help to increase circulation in the lower body, which helps to promote overall health and well-being. Seniors can stimulate blood flow to the muscles and tissues of the lower body, improving oxygenation and nutrient delivery, by swinging the leg forward, back, and side to side.

Lower Risk of Injury: Leg swings can help lower the risk of injury during physical activity by warming up the lower body's muscles and joints. This is crucial for seniors over 60 because they may be more prone to injuries or may require longer recovery periods after an injury.

How to Swing Your Legs Effectively and Safely

Follow these steps to do leg swings:

-With your hands on your hips or holding onto a chair or wall for support, stand with your feet hip-width apart.

-To keep your upper body stable and under control, contract your core muscles.

-Leaning slightly, shift your weight to your left leg.

-Straighten out your right leg as you swing it forward until it is parallel to the ground. Hold for a short while, then swing it as far as you can comfortably behind your body. Ten to fifteen times should be repeated with this motion.

-Next, extend your right leg to the side while maintaining its straightness until it is parallel to the ground. Hold for a short while, then swing it back in as far as you can comfortably across your body. Ten to fifteen times should be repeated with this motion.

-Replicate the exercise on the other side while switching legs.

Advice for Increasing the Difficulty of Leg Swings

Here are some ideas for making leg swings more difficult if you find them to be too easy:

-Increase the range of motion by swinging your leg higher, farther in front and back, or from side to side to make leg swings more difficult.

-Add resistance: By adding resistance, such as ankle weights or a resistance band around your ankles, you can make leg swings harder.

-Increasing the speed will make the exercise more difficult if you are confident in your ability to control the movement and are at ease with it.

Mat Exercises

Pelvic Tilt

The pelvic tilt is a simple mat exercise that involves tilting the pelvis forward and back. This exercise is designed to strengthen the muscles of the lower back and abdominals, as well as improve overall posture and alignment.

Benefits of Pelvic Tilt for Seniors

Pelvic tilt is a low-impact exercise that can provide seniors with many health benefits, including:

Improved posture and alignment: Pelvic tilt can help to correct postural imbalances and improve spinal alignment, which can reduce the risk of back pain and improve overall mobility.

Strengthening of the core: Pelvic tilt engages the muscles of the core, including the lower back and abdominal muscles. By strengthening these muscles, seniors can improve their balance, stability, and overall physical health.

Increased flexibility: Pelvic tilt can help to increase the flexibility of the lower back, hip flexors, and hamstrings. This can improve range of motion and reduce the risk of injury.

Improved Balance: Pelvic tilt requires balance and coordination, making it a great exercise for seniors who want to improve their balance and prevent falls.

How to Do Pelvic Tilt Exercise

To perform the pelvic tilt, follow these steps:

-Lie on your back on a mat with your knees bent and feet flat on the floor.

-Relax your shoulders and keep your arms at your sides.

-Begin by flattening your lower back against the mat. To do this, engage your abdominal muscles and press your lower back into the mat.

Hold this position for a few seconds, then release and allow your lower back to return to its natural curve.

-Next, arch your lower back slightly away from the mat. To do this, engage your lower back muscles and lift your hips slightly off the mat.

Hold this position for a few seconds, then release and allow your lower back to return to its natural curve. Repeat 10 to 15 times.

Tips for Making Pelvic Tilt More Challenging

If you find that pelvic tilts are too easy, here are some tips for making the exercise more challenging:

Increase the range of motion: To make pelvic tilts more challenging, increase the range of motion by lifting your hips higher or arching your lower back more.

Add Resistance: You can also make pelvic tilts more challenging by adding resistance, such as a small exercise ball or a resistance band around your thighs.

Increase the Duration: If you are comfortable with the movement and have good control, you can increase the duration of the exercise by holding each position for longer periods of time.

Leg Circles

Leg circles are a great lower body exercise for senior citizens because they target the glutes, hips, thighs, and calves. This enhances mobility, stability, and balance, all of which are crucial for aging adults. Leg Circles encourage blood flow and flexibility in the legs, which can help reduce joint pain and stiffness.

Leg circles can also help with posture by strengthening the lower back muscles, which can stop the occurrence of a rounded or hunched spine. This exercise can also help the body's circulation, which can result in better overall health and energy levels.

How to Do Leg Circulations:

-Start by lying on your back on a mat with your arms by your sides to prepare for Leg Circles. Point your toes upward while maintaining straight, joined legs. After that, slowly lift your right leg off the ground while maintaining its straightness to keep your balance.

-When your leg is raised, start moving it in a circle by rotating your ankle and moving your leg after that. You should be able to feel your leg muscles contracting as you move around a circle that is about the size of a basketball.

-Turn around and repeat the exercise with your left leg after making several circles in one direction. Throughout the exercise, it's crucial to maintain slow, controlled movement while paying attention to your breathing.

<u>Variations for Various Ability Levels:</u>

Leg Circles can be adapted in a number of ways to make them more accessible for seniors who are new to Pilates or who have limited mobility. It may be simpler for instance to maintain balance and control if the head and shoulders are supported by a pillow during the exercise.

Alternately, knee bends can be used to perform the circles, which can help relieve lower back strain and make the exercise more bearable for people with stiff or painful joints. Seniors who struggle with balance can also do Leg Circles while clinging to a chair or other sturdy object for support.

Leg Circles can be performed in a variety of ways for seniors who are more experienced or who want to increase the difficulty of their workout. An alternative is to include ankle weights to up the exercise's resistance and intensity. Another option is to make the circles while balancing a small ball or other object between the legs. This can help to work the inner thigh muscles and make the exercise more challenging.

Single Leg Stretch

A common Pilates mat exercise called the single leg stretch is especially good for people over 60. The abdominal muscles are the focus of this exercise, which also increases flexibility and balance and can lessen joint stiffness and pain. In this article, we'll go over the advantages of the single leg stretch, how to do it, and variations for people with various levels of fitness.

Advantages of a single-leg stretch

For seniors, the single leg stretch is a great exercise because it strengthens the abdominal muscles, which are crucial for good posture, balance, and stability. Additionally, the exercise encourages flexibility in the muscles of the hips and legs, which can ease stiffness and joint pain.

In order for seniors to maintain their independence and mobility, performing Single Leg Stretch can also help to strengthen the entire body. This exercise can lower the risk of injury and help prevent falls by strengthening the muscles in the core.

How to Perform Single Leg Stretch:

-Begin by laying on your back on a mat with your knees bent and your feet flat on the ground to perform the single leg stretch. With your elbows pointing outward, keep your hands behind your head. Engage your abdominal muscles and lift your head, neck, and shoulders off the mat.

-Lift your right leg off the mat and extend it out at a 45-degree angle after engaging your core. At the same time, bring your left knee in close to your chest while grabbing your shin or knee with your hands. After a brief period of holding this position, switch legs by stretching out your left leg and drawing your right knee toward your chest.

-Keep your movements controlled and slow to complete the exercise successfully. Keep your attention on your breathing, taking in air as you change legs and exhaling as you maintain the posture. Keeping your shoulders loose and avoiding straining your neck or upper back are also crucial.

Variations for Various Ability Levels:

There are several ways to make Single Leg Stretch more accessible for seniors who are new to Pilates or who have limited mobility. It may be simpler for instance to maintain control and balance if the head and shoulders are supported by a pillow during the exercise.

As an alternative, the exercise can be done with the legs bent at a 90-degree angle, which can help relieve lower back pressure and make the exercise more comfortable for people with joint pain or stiffness. Seniors can also perform Single Leg Stretch with their head resting on the mat if they have trouble lifting their head and shoulders off the floor.

There are additional Single Leg Stretch variations that can be performed for seniors who are more experienced or who want to increase the difficulty of their exercise. An alternative is to include ankle weights to up the exercise's resistance and intensity. Another choice is to carry out the exercise while supporting a small ball or other object between the legs. This can help to activate the inner thigh muscles and make the exercise more challenging.

<u>Guidelines for a secure and efficient Single-Leg Stretch</u>

To perform Single Leg Stretch safely and effectively, it is important to keep the following tips in mind:

Focus on your core: To get the most benefit from Single Leg Stretch, focus on maintaining your core stability. You'll be able to maintain balance and control while doing this, and your core muscles will get a good workout.

Keep your movements slow and controlled: When performing the single leg stretch, it's critical to do so in order to avoid injury and make sure you're targeting the appropriate muscles.

Keep proper form: Maintain a relaxed posture and refrain from tensing your neck or upper back. Stop the exercise and see a doctor or physical therapist as soon as you experience any discomfort or pain.

Start with a few Repetitions: It is best to begin the Single Leg Stretch with a few repetitions and increase the number as you become more at ease and confident with the exercise. As a general rule, start with 5–10 times on each leg, and as you get stronger, increase the number.

When performing the Single Leg Stretch, pay attention to your body. If you feel any pain or discomfort, stop the exercise right away and take a break. If you are new to Pilates or have a pre-existing medical condition, it is especially important to pay attention to your body and avoid overexerting yourself.

Double Leg Stretch

The double leg stretch is a classic Pilates exercise that is especially beneficial for seniors over the age of 60. This exercise is intended to strengthen core muscles while also improving flexibility, balance, and coordination. This sub chapter will go over the benefits of the Double Leg Stretch, how to do it, and variations for different levels of ability.

Advantages for Double Leg Stretch:

-The Double Leg Stretch is an excellent exercise for seniors because it targets the abdominal muscles, which are important for maintaining good posture, balance, and stability.

-Double Leg Stretching can also help improve balance and coordination, which are important for seniors who want to maintain their independence and mobility. This exercise, by working the muscles in the core and lower body, can help prevent falls and reduce the risk of injury.

How to Do a Double Leg Stretch

-To begin the Double Leg Stretch, lie on your back on a mat with your arms at your sides. Maintain a tight grip on your legs and point your toes. Lift your head, neck, and shoulders off the mat by engaging your abdominal muscles.

-Inhale and extend both legs out in front of you, keeping them together and at a 45-degree angle to the mat, after engaging your core. At the same time, extend your arms over your head, parallel to the floor.

-Exhale and use your core muscles to lift both legs back towards your chest, hugging your knees to your chest while lowering your arms to your sides. Hold this position for a few seconds before inhaling and extending your legs out in front of you.

-To get the most out of the exercise, keep your movements slow and controlled. Concentrate on your breathing, inhaling as you extend your legs and exhaling as you draw them in towards your chest. It is also critical to maintain a relaxed posture and avoid straining your neck or upper back.

<u>Variations for Various Ability Levels</u>

The exercise can be performed with the head and shoulders propped up on a pillow, making control and balance easier to maintain.

The exercise can also be performed with the legs bent at a 90-degree angle, which can relieve pressure on the lower back and make the exercise more comfortable for those who suffer from joint pain or stiffness. Seniors who have difficulty lifting their heads and shoulders off the mat can do a Double Leg Stretch with their head resting on the mat.

There are variations of the Double Leg Stretch that can be performed by seniors who are more advanced or who want to add more challenge to their workout. One option is to add ankle weights to the exercise to increase the resistance and intensity. Another option is to do the exercise while holding a small ball or other prop between your legs, which will help engage the inner thigh muscles and make the exercise more difficult.

Tips for Performing a Safe and Effective Double Leg Stretch

To perform the Double Leg Stretch safely and effectively, keep the following tips in mind:

Engage your core: To get the most out of the Double Leg Stretch, keep your abdominal muscles engaged throughout the exercise. This will assist you in maintaining control and stability, as well as effectively working the muscles in your core.

Keep your movements slow and controlled: It is critical to move slowly and with control during Double Leg Stretch to avoid injury and to ensure that you are working the right muscles.

Maintain proper posture: Maintain a relaxed posture and avoid straining your neck or upper back. Stop exercising and rest if you experience any discomfort or pain in these areas.

Breathe deeply: It is critical to breathe deeply and evenly throughout the exercise in order to maintain proper form and get the most out of the Double Leg Stretch. Exhale as you bring your legs in towards your chest and inhale as you extend them.

If you are new to Pilates or have limited mobility, begin with a few repetitions of the Double Leg Stretch and gradually increase the number as you become more comfortable and confident with the exercise. As a general rule, start with 5-10 repetitions and gradually increase the number over time.

Pay Attention to your body: If you feel any pain or discomfort during the Double Leg Stretch, stop immediately and rest. It is critical to listen to your body and avoid overdoing it, especially if you are new to Pilates or have a pre-existing medical condition.

Scissors

Scissors is a mat exercise in Pilates that emphasizes the core muscles, including the abs, lower back, and hips. It is a terrific workout for seniors over 60 who wish to improve their posture, balance, and flexibility, and strengthen their core muscles. Scissors involves raising and lowering the legs in a scissor-like motion, which serves to stimulate the muscles in the lower body and enhance overall mobility.

In this sub chapter, we will investigate the benefits of Scissors for seniors over 60, present step-by-step directions for practicing the exercise, and offer advice for safe and effective execution.

Advantages of Scissors for Seniors over 60

Increases core strength: Scissors is a highly effective workout for building core strength and stability. By working the muscles in the abdomen, lower back, and hips, this exercise helps to improve posture and balance, which can lessen the risk of falls and injury.

Enhances flexibility: Scissors helps to enhance flexibility in the hips and lower back, which can help alleviate pain and stiffness in these regions. Increased flexibility can also make daily activities, such as getting up from a chair or bending down to pick something up, easier and more pleasant.

Tones the lower body: Scissors specifically targets the muscles in the lower body, including the quadriceps, hamstrings, and glutes. By training these muscles, adults over 60 can increase their overall strength and mobility, making it easier to conduct regular chores.

Improves circulation: Scissors involves rising and lowering the legs, which helps to promote blood flow and circulation to the lower body. This can help decrease swelling and inflammation in the legs and feet, and promote overall health and wellness.

Step-by-Step Instructions to Doing Scissors

-Lay on your back with your legs stretched out and arms at your sides. Engage your core muscles by pulling your navel in towards your spine.

-Raise your legs off the mat, keeping them straight and together. Raise them towards the ceiling, until they are at a 90-degree angle with your torso.

-Drop your right leg towards the mat, while maintaining your left leg raised. Do not let your lower back lift off the mat.

-Keep your left leg in place and switch legs, elevating your right leg and lowering your left leg towards the mat.

-Repeat swapping legs in a scissor-like motion for 5-10 repetitions.

Recommendations for Safe and Efficient Execution

Engage your core: To execute Scissors safely and successfully, it is vital to activate your core muscles throughout the exercise. This helps to stabilize your lower back and pelvis and prevent damage.

Keep your legs straight: It is vital to keep your legs straight during Scissors, to optimize the involvement of the muscles in the lower body. If you have insufficient flexibility, you can adapt the workout by bending your knees slightly.

Do not elevate your lower back: As you lower one leg towards the ground, it is crucial to keep your lower back firmly planted against the mat. This helps to prevent strain on the lower back and maintain good form.

Breathe deeply: To get the most out of Scissors, it is crucial to breathe deeply and evenly during the exercise. Inhale as you swap legs and exhale as you hold your leg in place.

Start slowly and gradually build intensity: If you are new to Pilates or have restricted mobility, start with a few repetitions of Scissors and gradually raise the number as you feel more comfortable and confident with the exercise. As a general rule, attempt to accomplish 5-10 repetitions to start, and then steadily increase the number over time.

Listen to your body: If you suffer any pain or discomfort during the activity, stop immediately and consult with your healthcare professional before restarting.

Versions of Scissors

Reverse Scissors: This form of Scissors entails dropping both legs towards the mat, one at a time, and then lifting them back up to the beginning position. This is a more advanced variant that demands higher strength and stability.

Bicycle Scissors: Bicycle Scissors combines mixing Scissors with the Bicycle workout. Start in the Scissors position, and then pull your right knee towards your chest while straightening your left leg towards the ceiling. Switch legs, bringing your left knee towards your chest and straightening your right leg towards the ceiling. Continue swapping legs in a bicycle-like motion for 5-10 repetitions.

Open Leg Scissors: Open Leg Scissors includes opening your legs into a broad V-shape before switching them in a scissor-like action. This version adds an added challenge to the exercise by targeting the inner thighs.

Hip Circles

An abdominal, lower back, and hip-focused mat exercise is called a hip circle. Your knees should be bent and your feet should be flat on the floor while you practice this exercise while lying on your back on a mat. The exercise is rotating your hips in a circular manner to produce a soft, flowing action that aims to increase hip flexibility and mobility while also strengthening your lower body and core.

Advantages of Hip circles for Seniors

For several reasons, hip circles are a fantastic workout for Seniors, such exercises include:

Increased Hip Mobility: Our hips tend to become less mobile as we age, which can cause stiffness and discomfort. Hip circles can aid in enhancing hip mobility and lowering the risk of associated diseases like hip discomfort.

Hip circles are an excellent exercise for developing the core and lower body since they work the muscles in the lower back, hips, and thighs as well as the abdomen and lower back.

Decreased risk of falls: Hip circles can help lower the risk of falls and injuries by enhancing mobility, balance, and coordination, which can be crucial for seniors.

Decreased stress: The hip circles' soft, gliding motion can aid in reducing physical stress and tension and encouraging peace and relaxation.

How to work out Your Hip Circles Safely and Effortlessly

Follow these methods to execute hip circles exercise safely and effectively

-With your knees bent and your feet flat, lie on your back on a mat.

-With your hands down, position your arms at your sides.

-Take a deep breath in, contract your abdominal muscles, and press your lower back firmly into the mat as you exhale.

-Raise your hips off the mat so that your body forms a bridge shape. Keep your feet flat on the ground and your knees bent.

-Start rotating your hips in a circular manner to the right and then to the left once you are in the bridge position.

-Focus on tightening your abs and maintaining controlled, fluid movements as you circle your hips. The practice should be repeated 8 to 10 times.

Guidelines for Properly Doing the Hip Circles Workout

Follow these guidelines to practice hip circles safely:

-Keep your motions controlled and fluid: Avoid jerky or quick movements because they can lead to more injuries.

-Keep your attention on your breathing as you work out. As you lift your hips and circle them, inhale deeply and regularly.

-Do not strain your neck: Throughout the workout, keep your head and neck relaxed. Do not strain your neck by looking up or down.

-If necessary, lay a pillow or cushion beneath your lower back to support it during the workout if you have back pain or discomfort.

-To avoid overdoing it, stop exercising as soon as you experience any pain or discomfort and take a break. Don't exert too much effort.

Bridging

For seniors, bridging is a great mat exercise in Pilates. This exercise strengthens the muscles that support the spine and enhances mobility because it concentrates on the glutes, hamstrings, and lower back. Bridging can also aid with flexibility, coordination, and balance. We'll examine the advantages of bridging for seniors over 60 in this post and offer advice on good form and technique.

Guidelines for the Bridging Exercise

Make sure to warm up thoroughly before bridging by engaging in some modest cardiovascular exercise or stretching. When you're prepared to start, adhere to these guidelines:

-Your feet should be flat on the floor as you lay on your back with your knees bent. Your arms should be at your sides, and your feet should be hip-width apart.

-To lift your hips off the ground, plant your feet firmly on the ground and tighten your hamstrings and glutes. Your hips, shoulders, and knees ought to be in a straight line.

-After briefly maintaining the bridge position, bring your hips back down to the floor. Repeat 10 to 12 times altogether.

Advice on Form and Technique

Follow these guidelines for appropriate form and technique to make sure you get the most out of your bridging exercise and prevent injury:

-Draw your belly button toward your spine to activate your core before rising your hips. By doing so, you'll protect your lower back and make sure the exercise is being performed with the right muscles.

-Maintain Your Feet Parallel: Throughout the workout, keep your feet parallel and hip-width apart. By doing this, you'll be able to avoid having your knees fall inward or outward, which could put undue strain on the joints.

-Keep your Hips Level: Keep your hips level as you elevate them. It's best to prevent one hip from rising higher than the other because this can cause imbalances and uneven muscle growth.

-Don't Rush: When executing the workout, take your time and do not rush through the repetitions. Keep your form in check and use the appropriate muscles for each repetition.

-Breathe properly by inhaling before lifting your hips and exhaling as you do so. You'll be able to work your glutes and core more effectively as a result of this.

-Prevent Overexertion: Although it's crucial to push yourself during the workout, it's equally crucial to avoid overexertion. If you develop any symptoms of exhaustion, such as lightheadedness or breathing difficulty please stop.

Bridge Benefits for Seniors Over 60

Bridging has many physical and mental advantages, making it a great exercise for adults over 60. The following are a few advantages of bridging:

Strengthens Core Muscles: Bridging is a terrific approach to build the core muscles, which include the lower back, obliques, and abdominals. Maintaining balance and stability, which grow more crucial as we age, requires a strong core.

Enhances Posture: Bridging can assist to enhance posture and lower the chance of developing spinal abnormalities by strengthening the muscles that support the spine.

Reduces Lower Back Pain: By bolstering the muscles that support the spine, bridging helps reduce lower back discomfort. This may result in less pain and discomfort, which will make it simpler to go about your everyday business.

Enhances Flexibility: Seniors who may be experiencing stiffness and joint pain may find that bridging helps to increase their hips' range of motion and flexibility.

Enhances Balance and Coordination: Bridging calls for a lot of balance and coordination, which can aid in their improvement. Given that falls are one of the leading causes of injuries and disabilities in this demographic, seniors may benefit particularly from this.

Building muscle strength: Bridging focuses on the lower back, hamstrings, and glutes, which are all crucial muscle groups for preserving independence and mobility as we age.

Increases Bone Density: Research has shown that resistance training, such as bridging, increases bone density, which can help prevent osteoporosis and lower the risk of fractures.

Exercise has been demonstrated to alleviate stress and anxiety by generating endorphins, the body's naturally occurring feel-good hormones. Seniors' mental and emotional health can be greatly enhanced through bridging.

Safety Measures for Exercise in Bridge

Although bridging is generally risk-free for seniors over 60, there are a few safety measures that need to be followed to prevent harm. When practicing bridging, keep the following safety measures in mind:

Contact a doctor: To make sure you're healthy enough to participate in any new workout program, it's important to consult a doctor before beginning it.

Start Slowly: It's vital to start slowly and build up to more repetitions or sets if you're new to bridging or haven't worked out in a while.

Employ Correct Form: When executing bridging, be sure to use proper form and technique to avoid injury.

Don't Overexert Yourself: While pushing yourself during the workout is necessary, it's also crucial to avoid exhausting yourself too much. Stop the workout as soon as you feel any pain or discomfort.

Change the Exercise: You might need to change the exercise to fit your needs if you have any health issues or physical restrictions. To support your lower back, for instance, you might need to utilize a cushion or yoga block.

Spine Stretch

The spine stretch is a mat workout that involves stretching your spine forward while sitting with your legs straight in front of you. By increasing spine flexibility and mobility, this exercise helps lower the chance of developing back pain and other spinal problems. The abdominal muscles, which are crucial for preserving core strength and stability, are also worked by the spine stretch.

Advantages of Spine stretches for seniors over 60

The spine stretch is a great workout for seniors over 60 since it provides many significant advantages, such as:

Better Flexibility: The spine stretch is intended to increase spinal flexibility and mobility, which can help seniors retain their range of motion as they age.

Reduced Risk of Back Pain: The spine stretch can help to lower the risk of back pain and other spinal problems by strengthening the muscles that support the spine.

Better Posture: The spine stretch can help older adults stand taller and straighter by stretching the muscles in their backs and necks.

Strengthened Abdominal Muscles: The stretch of the spine also engages the abdominal muscles, which are crucial for preserving stability and core strength.

Reduction of Stress: The spine stretch is a calming exercise that can aid in lowering mental and physical strain.

How to Do the Workout to Stretch Your Spine

Observe these steps to safely and properly complete the spine stretch exercise:

-Legs straight out in front of you and shoulder-width apart as you sit on the mat.

-With your palms down, keep your arms straight and parallel to your legs.

-Taking a deep breath, extend your spine.

-Slowly exhale while extending your spine forward and touching your toes. While you stretch, keep your chin tucked down toward your chest.

-After a brief period of holding the stretch, inhale and slowly return to the beginning position. 5–10 times should be spent repeating the stretch.

Guidelines for Properly Doing the Spine Stretch

Follow these guidelines to safely conduct the spine stretch

Employ proper form: As you extend forward, be sure to maintain a straight back and relaxed shoulders. Do not put pressure on your neck nor your back.

Stretch Gradually: Don't bounce or jerk as you extend forward take your time.

Avoid Overdoing It: Stop the workout right away if you feel any pain or discomfort. Don't exert too much effort.

Change the Workout if Necessary: You might need to alter the exercise to fit your needs if you have any medical issues or physical restrictions. To support your lower back, for instance, you might need to utilize a cushion or yoga block.

Breathe deeply: Throughout the exercise, be careful to breathe deeply and rhythmically. Exhale slowly as you stretch forward while taking a deep breath to lengthen your spine.

Standing Exercises

Wall Roll-Down

In the standing exercise known as the "Wall Roll-Down," each vertebra of the spine is rolled down the wall one at a time. This exercise assists in lengthening the spine, enhancing posture, and easing neck and back strain. Another excellent exercise for developing balance and strengthening the core is the wall roll-down.

Wall Roll-Down Benefits for Seniors Over 60

For several reasons, including the following, the wall roll-down is a fantastic workout for seniors over 60.

Increased Flexibility: Our bodies tend to become less flexible as we become older. The back and spine's flexibility can be improved by wall roll-down, which lowers the risk of back discomfort and other related diseases.

Strengthened core and improved balance: The wall roll-down is an excellent workout for seniors since it works the core muscles and enhances balance.

Better posture: Wall Roll-Down can assist to improve posture and lower the risk of linked disorders including poor balance and falls by extending the spine and releasing tension in the back and neck.

Decreased stress: The Wall Roll-Down is a mild, fluid workout that can aid in reducing physical stress and tension while encouraging calm and relaxation.

How to Safely and Successfully Perform the Wall Roll-Down Workout

Follow these steps to safely and effectively complete the wall roll-down exercise.

-With your feet hip-width apart, stand with your back to a wall.

-Engage your abdominals while pushing your shoulders down and back.

-Inhale deeply, then start to roll your spine down the wall one vertebra at a time as you exhale.

-When you roll down, keep your knees slightly bent and let your head hang down toward the floor.

-Roll down as far as you can while still feeling comfortable, then hold the position for a few seconds.

-Take a deep breath in and start rolling your spine back up the wall one vertebra at a time as you exhale.

-Throughout the workout, keep your abs tight and your shoulders back and down. The practice should be repeated 8 to 10 times.

Guidelines for Properly Doing the Wall Roll-Down Workout

Consider the following advice to properly conduct the wall roll-down exercise:

-Keep your motions controlled and fluid: Avoid jerky or quick movements because they can lead to more injuries.

-Keep your attention on your breathing as you complete the exercise, inhaling and exhaling deeply and rhythmically as you roll down and up.

-Don't push yourself: If you experience any pain or discomfort, don't push yourself to move. Just descend the wall as far as you can comfortably.

-Keep your shoulders down: In order to preserve appropriate posture while you roll down the wall, keep your shoulders down.

-Keep your head and neck relaxed the entire time you are performing the exercise, and be careful not to overextend your neck when you roll down.

Leg Press

Leg press exercises on Pilates are a terrific approach for adults over 60 to increase their strength, balance, and general fitness. As we age, it becomes increasingly vital to maintain our muscular mass and strength, since this can help reduce falls and accidents, enhance mobility, and promote a better quality of life. Leg press exercises on Pilates can assist reach all of these aims, while also delivering a low-impact, safe workout that is accessible to seniors of all fitness levels.

In this sub chapter, we will discuss the benefits of leg press exercises on Pilates for seniors over 60, as well as providing suggestions and instructions for executing these exercises safely and successfully.

Benefits of Leg Press Exercises on Pilates for Seniors

Enhanced Strength

Leg press exercises on Pilates are an excellent approach to develop strength in the lower body, including the quadriceps, hamstrings, glutes, and calves. This can allow elders to conduct daily activities more effortlessly, such as climbing stairs, getting up from a chair, and walking.

Better Balance

As we age, our balance tends to diminish, which can increase the risk of falls and injuries. Leg press exercises on Pilates can assist improve balance by strengthening the muscles in the lower body, as well as the core muscles that are necessary for maintaining stability.

Low-Impact Exercise

Many seniors may have joint discomfort or other health issues that make high-impact workouts difficult or painful. Leg press exercises on Pilates are a low-impact alternative that can deliver many of the same benefits as high-impact workouts, without putting excessive strain on the joints.

Improved Bone Density

Weight-bearing activities, such as leg press exercises on Pilates, can help enhance bone density and minimize the risk of osteoporosis. This is particularly crucial for elderly, as the risk of osteoporosis grows with age.

Better Mood and Mental Health

Exercise has been found to promote mood and mental health, and leg press exercises on Pilates are no exception. Seniors who engage in regular exercise may report lower rates of depression, anxiety, and other mental health disorders.

Tips for Doing Leg Press Exercises on Pilates Safely and Successfully

Start Gently and Build Up Gradually

It's crucial for seniors to start cautiously and build up gradually when completing leg press exercises on Pilates. This will assist prevent injuries and guarantee that the exercises are successful. Seniors should begin with a low weight or resistance, then gradually raise the weight or resistance as they become stronger and more comfortable with the exercises.

Use Correct Form

Correct technique is vital for gaining the most benefit from leg press exercises on Pilates, as well as for preventing injuries. Seniors should make sure to keep their feet flat on the footplate and their knees in line with their toes. They should also avoid locking their knees at the height of the action, as this might place additional strain on the joints.

Use a Spotter

Seniors who are new to leg press exercises on Pilates or who are lifting high weights should employ a spotter to verify that they are utilizing good technique and to prevent accidents. A spotter can also provide support and encouragement during the activity.

Consult a Doctor

Seniors with health concerns or who are taking medication should check their doctor before beginning any new fitness program, including leg press exercises on Pilates. This will help guarantee that they are healthy enough to partake in the workouts and that there are no hazards or consequences.

Warm Up and Cool Down

Warming up and cooling down are key for preventing injuries and receiving the maximum benefit from leg press exercises on Pilates. Seniors should begin each activity with a few minutes of easy cardio, such as walking or cycling, and some dynamic stretching to prepare their muscles and joints for the activities. After the activity, kids should spend a few minutes cooling down with some static stretching to help avoid muscular tightness and increase flexibility.

Examples of Leg Press Exercises on Pilates for Seniors

Basic Leg Press

The basic leg press is a fantastic exercise for seniors to begin with, as it is easy and low-impact. To complete this exercise, seniors should sit on the Pilates machine with their back against the backrest and their feet on the footplate. They should then push the footplate away from them, extending their legs until they are straight. They should then carefully lower the footplate back to the beginning position, bending their knees as they do so.

Single Leg Press

The single leg press is a variation of the basic leg press that can help improve balance and stability. To perform this exercise, seniors should sit on the Pilates machine with one foot on the footplate and the other foot on the floor. They should then push the footplate away from them, extending their leg until it is straight. They should then slowly lower the footplate back to the starting position, bending their knee as they do so. They should then repeat the exercise with the other leg.

Calf Raises

Calf raises are a terrific approach to strengthen the calf muscles, which are vital for balance and stability. To execute this exercise, elders should sit on the Pilates machine with their feet on the footplate. They should then push the footplate away from them, extending their legs until they are straight. They should next lift their heels off the footplate, lifting their bodies up on their toes. They should then progressively lower their heels back to the beginning position.

Hip Abduction

Hip abduction is an excellent exercise for developing the glutes and outer thighs, which are vital for stability and balance. To execute this exercise, elders should sit on the Pilates machine with their feet on the footplate. They should then push the footplate away from them, extending their legs until they are straight. They should then open their legs out to the sides, maintaining their feet flat on the footplate. They should then carefully draw their legs back together.

Leg Curl

Leg curl workouts primarily target the hamstrings, which are vital muscles for walking and standing. In this post, we will investigate the benefits of leg curl exercises on Pilates for seniors over 60, as well as providing recommendations for executing these exercises safely and successfully.

Advantages of Leg Curl Exercises on Pilates for Seniors over 60

Enhanced Muscular Strength

Leg curl exercises on Pilates can assist enhance the strength of the hamstrings, which are vital muscles for walking and standing. Strong hamstrings can help seniors keep their balance and reduce falls, which are common among older persons. By strengthening muscle strength, elders can also increase their mobility and independence.

Improved Bone Density

Weight-bearing activities, such as leg curl exercises, can help enhance bone density and reduce the risk of osteoporosis. Osteoporosis is a disorder in which the bones become weak and brittle, and is a prevalent concern among elderly persons. By completing leg curl movements on Pilates, elders can help strengthen their bones and prevent the chance of fractures.

Enhanced Flexibility

Leg curl exercises on Pilates can also help increase flexibility in the hamstrings and other lower body muscles.

Increased flexibility can help seniors move more smoothly and with less discomfort, and can also minimize the chance of muscular strains and other accidents.

Better Balance and Stability

Leg curl exercises on Pilates can assist improve balance and stability, which are vital for reducing falls and accidents. These exercises engage the muscles in the legs and hips, which are necessary for maintaining balance and stability while standing or walking. By increasing balance and stability, seniors can lower their risk of falls and injuries, which can have a substantial impact on their quality of life.

Tips for Doing Leg Curl Exercises on Pilates Safely and Effectively

Warm-Up and Stretch

Before completing leg curl exercises on Pilates, elders should warm up and stretch to prepare their muscles and joints. Active stretching, such as walking or light running, can assist boost blood flow and warm up the muscles. Static stretching, such as holding a stretch for 15-30 seconds, can assist increase flexibility and reduce the chance of injury.

Use Correct Form

When performing leg curl movements on Pilates, elders should utilize perfect technique to minimize injury and optimize the advantages of the exercise. They should keep their core engaged and their back upright, and avoid arching their back or leaning forward. They should also keep their knees in line with their ankles and avoid letting their knees turn inward or outward.

Utilize Appropriate Resistance

Seniors should utilize an appropriate level of resistance when conducting leg curl exercises on Pilates. They should start with a low resistance and progressively raise the resistance as they gain stronger. Applying too much resistance might put too much strain on the muscles and raise the chance of damage.

Breathe

Seniors should remember to breathe while completing leg curl movements on Pilates. They should inhale as they bend their knees and exhale as they straighten their legs. Breathing can aid enhance oxygen flow to the muscles and boost performance.

Examples of Leg Curl Exercises on Pilates for Senior

Simple Leg Curl

The fundamental leg curl is a simple and effective exercise for seniors to begin with. To complete this exercise, seniors should lie face down on the Pilates machine with their ankles hooked beneath the foot bar. They should then bend their knees, putting their heels nearer their buttocks. They should then carefully drop their legs back to the beginning position.

Standing Leg Curl

The Standing leg curl is a version of the basic leg curl that may be performed while standing up. To complete this exercise, elders should stand with their feet shoulder-width apart and place a resistance band around their ankles. They should next elevate one foot off the ground and bend their knee, bringing their heel toward their buttocks. They should then carefully lower their leg back to the beginning position and repeat with the other leg.

Seated Leg Curl

The seated leg curl is another variation of the standard leg curl that may be performed while sitting down. To complete this exercise, seniors should sit on the Pilates machine with their legs extended in front of them and their ankles hooked beneath the foot bar. They should then bend their knees, putting their heels nearer their buttocks. They should then carefully drop their legs back to the beginning position.

Single-Leg Deadlift

The single-leg deadlift is a more advanced leg curl exercise that can assist improve balance and stability. To complete this exercise, seniors should stand with their feet hip-width apart and grasp a dumbbell or kettlebell in their right hand. They should next lift their left foot off the ground and stretch their left leg behind them, while bending forward at the waist and reducing the weight toward the ground. They should then return to the beginning position and repeat with the other leg.

Squat

Squats are a versatile and effective exercise that may be adapted to meet the demands of seniors over 60. Pilates is an ideal approach to incorporate squats into a senior's workout program, as Pilates stresses perfect form and alignment, which can help seniors perform squats safely and effectively. In this post, we will study numerous squat exercises on Pilates that are ideal for seniors over 60.

Basic Squat

The basic squat is a wonderful exercise to start with for seniors who are new to Pilates. To complete this exercise, elders should stand with their feet shoulder-width apart and their toes pointed forward. They should next bend their knees, keeping their heels on the ground, and lower their buttocks toward the earth. They should attempt to keep their back straight and their knees aligned with their toes. As they reach a comfortable depth, they should push through their heels and return to the beginning position.

Wall Squat

The wall squat is another wonderful version of the fundamental squat that may be performed by seniors. To complete this exercise, elders should stand with their back against a wall and their feet hip-width apart. They should then slowly drop their butts toward the ground while sliding down the wall, as if they are sitting in an imaginary chair. They should attempt to keep their knees aligned with their toes and their back flat on the wall. As they reach a comfortable depth, they should push through their heels and return to the beginning position.

Single-Leg Squat

The single-leg squat is a more advanced squat exercise that can help improve balance and stability. To complete this exercise, seniors should stand on one leg and elevate the other leg off the ground. They should then slowly drop their buttocks toward the ground while keeping their elevated leg extended in front of them. They should attempt to keep their back straight and their supporting knee aligned with their toes. As they reach a comfortable depth, they should push through their supporting heel and return to the starting position. They should then repeat the practice on the other leg.

Sumo Squat

The sumo squat is a modification of the standard squat that emphasizes the inner thigh muscles. To complete this exercise, elders should stand with their feet wider than shoulder-width apart and their toes pointing outward. They should next descend their buttocks toward the ground while keeping their back straight and their knees aligned with their toes. As they reach a comfortable depth, they should push through their heels and return to the beginning position.

Goblet Squat

The goblet squat is a variation of the standard squat that can be performed with a weight, such as a dumbbell or kettlebell. To complete this exercise, seniors should hold the weight at chest level with both hands and stand with their feet shoulder-width apart. They should next descend their buttocks toward the ground while keeping their back straight and their knees aligned with their toes. As they reach a comfortable depth, they should push through their heels and return to the beginning position.

Suggestions for Seniors

Seniors over 60 can take some care while performing squat exercises on Pilates to protect their safety and avoid injury. Here are some tips for seniors:

-Start with simple squats and graduate gradually to more advanced versions.

-Employ good form and alignment when executing the workout. Seniors should keep their back straight, their knees aligned with their toes, and their feet flat on the ground.

-Employ suitable resistance that challenges but does not strain the muscles. Seniors should start with smaller weights or resistance bands and build gradually over time.

-Integrate breathing techniques into the exercise. Seniors should inhale before they drop their buttocks and exhale as they push through their heels to return to the starting posture.

-Always warm up before beginning squat workouts. Seniors could engage some light aerobic exercise, like as walking or cycling, for a few minutes to boost their heart rate and increase blood flow to their muscles.

-Seniors should also stretch their muscles before and after the activity to prevent stiffness and pain. They should focus on stretching their quadriceps, hamstrings, and hip flexors.

Advantages of Squat Exercises for Seniors

Squat exercises on Pilates can provide various benefits for seniors over 60, including:

Increased Balance and Stability: Squat exercises demand seniors to activate their core and stabilizing muscles, which can assist improve their balance and stability. This can help lessen the risk of falls and injuries.

Stronger leg muscles: Squat workouts target the quadriceps, hamstrings, and gluteal muscles, which can help strengthen the legs and increase mobility.

Increased joint health: Squat exercises can assist improve joint health by boosting the generation of synovial fluid, which lubricates the joints and minimizes friction.

Improved bone density: Squat workouts can help increase bone density, which can help avoid osteoporosis and fractures.

Increased cardiovascular health: Squat workouts can assist enhance cardiovascular health by boosting the heart rate and increasing blood supply to the muscles.

Calf Raises

Calf raises are a basic workout in which you stand on your toes and elevate your heels off the ground. This exercise works the calf muscles, particularly the gastrocnemius and soleus. Calf raises can be done with your own weight or with the help of dumbbells, resistance bands, or a machine.

The Advantages of Calf Raises for Elderly Over 60

Calf raises provide various advantages to seniors over the age of 60, including:

-Increased balance*:* Calf muscle strength is essential for balance, which can help prevent falls and other injuries.

-Increased mobility: Strong calf muscles can help with movement and make daily activities like walking and climbing stairs easier.

-Calf raises can enhance circulation in the lower legs, lowering the risk of blood clots and other circulation-related disorders.

-Weight-bearing workouts such as calf raises can enhance bone density and lower the risk of osteoporosis.

-Calf raises are a low-impact activity, which means they are less likely to produce joint pain or damage than high-impact exercises such as jogging or jumping.

Adding Calf Raises to a Senior's Workout Program

Calf raises can be included into a senior's workout routine in a variety of ways. Calf raises on a machine at a gym or fitness center are one alternative. Another option is to do calf raises at home using dumbbells, resistance bands, or other equipment.

-Calf raises should be performed 2-3 times per week by seniors, beginning with 1-2 sets of 8-12 repetitions. They can gradually raise the weight or resistance level, as well as the number of sets and repetitions, as their strength and comfort level improve.

-Calf raises should be part of a full-body fitness plan that that includes stretching, balance exercises, and cardio. Before beginning any new exercise program, seniors should speak with a doctor or physical therapist, especially if they have a history of joint difficulties or other health issues.

Pilates Techniques for Calf Raises

To get the most out of calf raises, make sure you practice appropriate technique and avoid common mistakes. Here are some pointers for performing calf lifts on the Pilates mat:

-Stand shoulder-width apart with your feet shoulder-width apart and your toes pointed forward.

-Gently rise up onto the balls of your feet, elevating your heels as high off the ground as possible.

-Maintain the top position for a few seconds before slowly lowering your heels to the ground.

-Throughout the workout, keep your core engaged and your posture upright. Elevate your heels off the ground, avoid bouncing or using momentum to avoid damage, keep your movements calm and controlled.

Cool-Down Exercises

Seated Forward Fold

A seated forward fold is a yoga and Pilates exercise that stretches the hamstrings, lower back, and neck muscles. This exercise involves sitting with your legs straight out in front of you and slowly folding forward, reaching toward your toes. This stretch can be modified to accommodate different flexibility levels by using props like a yoga strap or bolster.

Benefits of Seated Forward Folds for Seniors Over 60

Seated forward folds offer several benefits for seniors over 60, including:

Improved flexibility: Seated forward folds can improve flexibility in the hamstrings, lower back, and neck muscles, which can improve posture and reduce the risk of injury.

Reduced Tension: This stretch can relieve tension in the lower back and neck muscles, which can reduce pain and discomfort.

Improved Digestion: Forward folds can stimulate the digestive system and promote healthy digestion.

Improved Circulation: Seated forward folds can improve circulation in the lower body, which can reduce the risk of blood clots and other circulation-related issues.

Incorporating Seated Forward Folds into a Senior's Exercise Routine

Seniors can incorporate seated forward folds into their exercise routine by performing them as a cool-down exercise after a Pilates workout. This stretch can also be performed at home, either on a mat or in a chair, using props like a yoga strap or bolster to accommodate different flexibility levels.

Seniors should aim to hold the stretch for 30-60 seconds, breathing deeply and slowly throughout the stretch. They can repeat the stretch 1-3 times, depending on their comfort level and flexibility.

It's important to note that seniors should listen to their bodies and avoid over-stretching or pushing themselves too hard. If they experience pain or discomfort during the stretch, they should ease up or modify the stretch using props.

Tips for Performing Seated Forward Folds on Pilates

To get the most benefit from seated forward folds, it's important to use proper technique and avoid common mistakes. Here are some tips for performing seated forward folds on Pilates:

-Sit with your legs straight out in front of you, with your feet flexed and your toes pointing up.

-Inhale deeply, reaching your arms up overhead.

-Exhale slowly, folding forward from your hips, reaching your arms toward your toes.

-Keep your spine straight and your shoulders relaxed throughout the stretch. Hold the stretch for 30-60 seconds, breathing deeply and slowly. To release the stretch, inhale deeply, and slowly roll back up to a seated position.

-Use props like a yoga strap or bolster to modify the stretch if needed.

Hip Flexor Stretch

Hip flexors are a collection of muscles that are involved for flexing the hip joint and are frequently stiff in seniors as a result of a sedentary lifestyle. In this post, we will look at the benefits of hip flexor stretches as Pilates cool-down exercises for seniors over 60, as well as some recommendations for doing them safely and successfully.

Hip Flexor Stretches as Pilates Cool-Down Exercises for Seniors Over 60

Hip flexor stretches can give a variety of benefits for adults over 60 who add them into their Pilates regimen as cool-down exercises, including:

Better Posture

Tight hip flexors can tilt the pelvis forward, resulting in bad posture. Stretching the hip flexors can assist to release these muscles and improve posture, which can relieve back discomfort and increase general mobility.

Injury risk is reduced.

Tight hip flexors can also increase the risk of injury, especially in the lower back and knees. Regular stretching of these muscles can assist to prevent injury by improving flexibility and mobility.

Enhanced mobility

Our joints and muscles stiffen as we age, limiting our mobility. Hip flexor stretches can help to improve hip flexibility and mobility, allowing for a wider range of motion.

Reduction of Hip Pain

Stiff hip flexors can cause hip and lower back pain. Stretching these muscles can help relieve pain and stiffness, allowing seniors to do daily tasks more easily.

Better Circulation.

Stretching the hip flexors can also aid to enhance circulation, particularly in the legs. This can aid in the reduction of edema and the overall improvement of cardiovascular health.

Hip Flexor Stretches as Pilates Cool-Down Exercises for Seniors Over 60

These are several hip flexor stretches that are appropriate as Pilates cool-down exercises for seniors over 60:

Lunge at a Low Level

The low lunge is an excellent hip flexor stretch that may be done on a mat or a towel. Here's how to go about it:

-Begin by kneeling with your hands on your hips.

-Stride forward with your left foot, bending your left knee to a 90-degree angle. Maintain your right knee on the ground.

-Feel the stretch in your right hip flexor as you press your hips forward and down.

-Hold the stretch for 15-30 seconds before releasing it and switching sides.

Posture of a Pigeon

Another powerful hip flexor stretch that may be done on a mat or a towel is the pigeon stance. Here's how to go about it:

-Begin on your hands and knees on a tabletop.

-Move your right knee forward and behind your right hand.

-Stretch your left leg behind you, toes tucked underneath.

-Lower your body to the ground slowly, experiencing the stretch in your right hip flexor.

-Hold the stretch for 15-30 seconds before releasing it and switching sides.

Butterfly Stretch While Sitting

The seated butterfly stretch is a simple hip flexor stretch that you can do while sitting on a mat or towel. Here's how to go about it:

-Sit on the ground with your knees bent and your soles touching.

-Hands on your ankles or feet, gently press your knees down towards the earth.

-Maintain a straight back and Hold the stretch for 15-30 seconds.

Quad Stretch While Standing

Standing quad stretches are a basic yet effective hip flexor stretch that may be done while standing. Here's how to go about it:

-Place your feet shoulder-width apart.

-Raise your right foot off the ground and pull it towards your buttocks, your right hand gripping your ankle.

-Maintain a straight back and a slightly bent left knee.

-Hold the stretch for 15-30 seconds before releasing it and switching sides.

How to Do Hip Flexor Stretches Safely and Successfully

It is critical to execute hip flexor stretches as cool-down exercises for Pilates for seniors over 60 in a safe and effective manner. These are some pointers to remember:

-Begin slowly and progressively increase the intensity.

Begin with moderate stretches and progressively increase the intensity over time. This will aid in injury prevention and allow the body to acclimatize to the stretches.

-Pay attention to your body.

Take note of how your body feels during the stretches. Stop the stretch and adjust as needed if you suffer pain or discomfort.

-Make use of props.

Props like as a mat, towel, or yoga block can be used to support the body and make stretches more accessible.

-Include stretching in your everyday regimen.

Stretching should be incorporated into your everyday practice to preserve flexibility and mobility. Stretching can be done in the morning, before activity, or before bed.

Modified Exercises for Common Issues

Arthritis

Arthritis is a prevalent ailment that affects a large number of seniors over the age of 60. It can cause discomfort, stiffness, and decreased mobility, making physical activities like Pilates difficult to do. Pilates, with some changes, can be a safe and effective workout alternative for seniors suffering from arthritis. This sub chapter will go over adapted movements for common arthritis difficulties in Pilates for seniors over 60.

What exactly is arthritis?

Arthritis is a condition that affects the joints, causing inflammation and pain. There are many different varieties of arthritis, but the two most frequent in seniors are osteoarthritis and rheumatoid arthritis. Rheumatoid arthritis is an inflammatory illness that assaults the joints, whereas osteoarthritis occurs when the cartilage that cushions the joints wears down over time.

Pilates for Arthritic Seniors

Pilates is a low-impact workout that emphasizes core strength, flexibility, and balance. It can be an excellent kind of exercise for seniors with arthritis since it strengthens the muscles surrounding the joints, enhancing support and lowering pain. Certain adaptations may be required, however, to make Pilates safe and comfortable for persons with arthritis.

Adapted Exercises for Common Arthritis Problems

Knee Problems

Knee arthritis can cause discomfort and stiffness in the joint, making it difficult to execute exercises that require bending or twisting of the knee. Try the following modifications to Pilates routines for knee arthritis:

Exercises that require extensive knee bending or twisting, such as the kneeling lunge or roll-up, should be avoided.

Place a small pillow or folded towel between the knees for support during the Pilates bridge practice.

Perform the Pilates leg circles exercise lying on your back, with your affected knee bent and your foot on the ground.

Hip Problems

Hip arthritis can cause joint pain and stiffness, making it difficult to do movements that require hip flexion or rotation. Try the following modifications to Pilates routines for hip arthritis:

Exercises that demand considerable hip flexion or rotation, such as the Pilates bicycle or crisscross, should be avoided.

To add support to the Pilates hip bridge exercise, place a small cushion or folded towel between the knees.

Attempt the Pilates side-lying leg lift exercise, which focuses on engaging the hip and thigh muscles.

Shoulder Problems

Shoulder arthritis can cause joint pain and stiffness, making it difficult to execute workouts that require lifting or reaching. Try the following modifications to Pilates routines for shoulder arthritis:

Exercises that require lifting or reaching overhead, such as the Pilates overhead press or push-up, should be avoided.

Do the Pilates plank exercise on your forearms rather than your hands.

Attempt the Pilates chest opener exercise, which focuses on stretching and opening the shoulders.

Wrist Problems

Wrist arthritis can cause joint pain and stiffness, making it difficult to do exercises requiring grasping or bearing weight on the hands. Try the following modifications to Pilates routines for wrist arthritis:

Exercises requiring considerable gripping or bearing weight on the hands, such as the Pilates push-up or plank, should be avoided.

Place the injured arm on a small pillow or folded towel for support during the Pilates side-lying leg lift exercise.

Attempt the Pilates spine stretch forward exercise, which focuses on extending and working the core muscles.

Pilates Exercises Recommendations for Seniors with Arthritis

There are some general recommendations that can help make Pilates safe and successful for seniors with arthritis, in addition to adapted exercises:

Warm Up Before Beginning Pilates

Warming up before beginning Pilates is critical to reducing the chance of injury and improving flexibility. Walking, cycling, or stretching exercises are examples of gentle warm-up activities.

Employ props to help you.

Props such as cushions, blankets, or resistance bands can give support and alleviate joint tension. Placing a pillow between the knees during the Pilates bridge exercise, for example, can help to support the lower back and knees.

Concentrate on Alignment

Pilates requires precise alignment, which is especially important for seniors with arthritis. Concentrating on good alignment can help to reduce joint tension and increase the effectiveness of activities. Working with a trained Pilates instructor who can help you through the right alignment for each exercise is essential.

The importance of consistency

When it comes to Pilates for seniors with arthritis, consistency is crucial. It is critical to set and stick to a regular Pilates regimen in order to reap the benefits of the workout. To avoid overexertion and injury, begin with shorter sessions and gradually increase the duration and intensity.

<u>Osteoporosis</u>

Osteoporosis is a medical disorder defined by a loss of bone density, which leads to weak bones and an increased risk of fractures. It affects both men and women, but it is more common in postmenopausal women because to the hormonal changes that occur after menopause. Exercise is an important element of controlling osteoporosis, since it can help strengthen bones, improve balance, and lower the risk of falls and fractures. Pilates is a low-impact kind of exercise that can be particularly good for seniors with osteoporosis, as it focuses on increasing strength, flexibility, and balance. Nonetheless, certain adaptations may need to be made to meet frequent difficulties in seniors with osteoporosis.

These are some adapted Pilates routines for frequent difficulties in seniors with osteoporosis:

Rounded Shoulders:

Many seniors with osteoporosis develop a rounded posture due to weakening back muscles. To address this issue, exercises that focus on strengthening the upper back muscles and opening up the chest can be effective. Some examples of modified Pilates movements for rounded shoulders include the seated row and the chest stretch.

Seated Row:

Sit on a mat with your legs straight out in front of you, a resistance band around your feet, and the band grasped in both hands. Draw the band back towards your chest, pulling your shoulder blades together as you do so. Release and repeat for 10-15 repetitions.

Chest Stretch:

Stand with your feet hip-distance apart and your arms out to the sides at shoulder height. Reach your right arm across your body, placing your hand on your left shoulder blade. Use your left hand to gently draw your right elbow towards your left shoulder. Hold for 15-30 seconds, then repeat on the opposite side.

Weak Hips:

Weak hip muscles can contribute to poor balance and an increased risk of falls. To alleviate this condition, activities that focus on strengthening the hip muscles can be effective. Some examples of modified Pilates exercises for weak hips include the sitting hip abduction and the seated hip extension.

Seated Hip Abduction:

Sit on a mat with your legs straight out in front of you and a resistance band around your ankles. Spread your legs out to the sides, keeping your knees straight. Hold for 2-3 seconds, then release and continue for 10-15 repetitions.

Seated Hip Extension:

Sit on a mat with your legs straight out in front of you and a resistance band around your ankles. Raise your right foot off the ground, keeping your knee straight, and extend your leg back behind you. Hold for 2-3 seconds, then release and continue for 10-15 repetitions on each leg.

Weak Ankles:

Weak ankles can contribute to poor balance and an increased risk of falls. To alleviate this condition, activities that focus on strengthening the ankle muscles can be effective. Some examples of modified Pilates movements for weak ankles include ankle circles and heel raises.

Ankle Circles:

Sit on a mat with your legs straight out in front of you and your feet flexed. Circle your ankles in one way for 10-15 repetitions, then reverse and circle in the other direction for 10-15 repetitions.

Heel Raises:

Stand with your feet hip-distance apart and your hands resting on a chair or wall for support. Raise your heels off the ground, coming up onto the balls of your feet. Hold for 2-3 seconds, then lower and continue for 10-15 repetitions.

Kyphosis:

Kyphosis is an excessive rounding of the upper spine, which can contribute to bad posture and back pain. To address this issue, activities that focus on strengthening the upper back muscles and improving posture can be effective. Some examples of modified Pilates exercises for kyphosis include the shoulder blade squeeze and the spine stretch forward.

Shoulder Blade Squeeze:

Sit on a mat with your legs straight out in front of you and your arms down by your sides. Pull your shoulder blades together, bringing them down towards your back pockets. Hold for 2-3 seconds, then release and continue for 10-15 repetitions.

Spine Stretch Forward:

Sit on a mat with your legs straight out in front of you and your arms extended out in front of you. Inhale, then exhale as you round your spine and stretch towards your toes. Hold for 2-3 seconds, then inhale and roll back up to a seated posture. Repeat for 5-10 repetitions.

Balance Issues:

Elderly with osteoporosis may be at an increased risk of falls due to balance concerns. To alleviate this condition, activities that focus on increasing balance can be effective. Some examples of modified Pilates exercises for balance concerns include the single-leg balancing and the toe taps.

Single-Leg Balance:

Stand with your feet hip-distance apart and your hands resting on a chair or wall for support. Raise one foot off the ground and balance on the other foot for 10-15 seconds, then swap sides and repeat.

Toe Taps:

Stand with your feet hip-distance apart and your hands resting on a chair or wall for support. Raise one foot off the ground and tap your toe on the ground in front of you, then tap it to the side, then tap it behind you. Repeat for 10-15 times on each foot.

It's crucial to emphasize that seniors with osteoporosis should always contact with their healthcare provider before starting any new fitness regimen, including Pilates. Moreover, alterations may need to be made on a case-by-case basis based on the severity of osteoporosis and any other medical issues present. With adequate coaching and adaptations, Pilates can be a safe and effective type of exercise for seniors with osteoporosis.

In addition to these adjusted exercises, seniors with osteoporosis may also benefit from engaging in Pilates sessions specifically suited for their needs. These sessions may contain additional modifications and adjustments to accommodate frequent difficulties among seniors with osteoporosis. Also, engaging with a competent Pilates instructor who has experience working with seniors with osteoporosis can help verify that exercises are being completed safely and successfully.

Back Pain

Back discomfort is a prevalent condition that affects many elderly. It can be caused by a multitude of reasons, including osteoporosis, spinal stenosis, arthritis, and degenerative disc disease. Pilates, a low-impact kind of exercise that focuses on improving strength, flexibility, and balance, can be a good form of exercise for seniors with back discomfort. Nonetheless, adaptations may need to be made to meet frequent concerns in seniors with back discomfort. These are some modified Pilates movements for frequent concerns in seniors with back pain:

Weak Core:

A weak core can lead to back discomfort, as it places extra stress on the spine. Pilates routines that focus on strengthening the core can help relieve back discomfort. Some examples of modified Pilates movements for a weak core include the pelvic tilt and the bird dog.

Pelvic Tilt:

Lay on your back with your legs bent and your feet flat on the ground. Inhale, then exhale as you gradually tilt your pelvis towards your belly button, flattening your lower back into the ground. Hold for 2-3 seconds, then release and continue for 10-15 times.

Bird Dog:

Begin on your hands and knees, with your wrists directly under your shoulders and your knees directly under your hips. Inhale, then exhale as you lift one arm and the opposing leg off the ground, stretching them straight out in front of you and behind you, respectively. Hold for 2-3 seconds, then release and repeat on the opposite side. Repeat for 5-10 times on both sides.

Rounded Shoulders:

Rounded shoulders can contribute to poor posture and back pain. Pilates routines that focus on opening up the chest and strengthening the upper back can assist improve posture and alleviate back discomfort. Some examples of modified Pilates movements for rounded shoulders include the chest opener and the shoulder blade squeeze.

Chest Opener:

Sit on a mat with your legs straight out in front of you and your arms spread out to the sides. Inhale, then exhale as you slowly twist your upper body to one side, reaching your opposing arm towards your toes and your other arm towards the ceiling. Hold for 2-3 seconds, then release and repeat on the opposite side. Repeat for 5-10 times.

Shoulder Blade Squeeze:

Sit on a mat with your legs straight out in front of you and your arms down by your sides. Pull your shoulder blades together, bringing them down towards your back pockets. Hold for 2-3 seconds, then release and continue for 10-15 repetitions.

Hip Weakness:

Weak hips can contribute to poor posture and back pain. Pilates routines that focus on strengthening the hips can assist improve posture and alleviate back discomfort. Some examples of modified Pilates exercises for hip weakness include the clamshell and the hip bridge.

Clamshell:

Lay on your side with your knees bent and your feet together. With your feet together, lift your top knee towards the ceiling, then lower it back down. Repeat for 10-15 repetitions on each side.

Hip Bridge:

Lay on your back with your knees bent and your feet flat on the ground. Inhale, then exhale as you lift your hips towards the ceiling, squeezing your glutes and engaging your core. Hold for 2-3 seconds, then release and continue for 10-15 repetitions.

Spinal Stenosis:

Spinal stenosis is a disorder that causes the spinal canal to narrow, exerting pressure on the spinal cord and nerves. Pilates movements that focus on opening up the spinal column can help alleviate pressure and relieve discomfort. Some examples of modified Pilates exercises for spinal stenosis include the cat stretch and the child's posture

Cat Stretch:

Begin on your hands and knees, with your wrists immediately under your shoulders and your knees directly under your hips. Inhale, then exhale as you curve your spine towards the ceiling, tucking your chin towards your chest. Hold for 2-3 seconds, then release and continue for 10-15 repetitions.

Child's Pose:

Begin on your hands and knees, with your wrists directly under your shoulders and your knees directly under your hips. Inhale, then exhale as you sit back towards your heels, stretching your arms out in front of you. Hold for 10-15 seconds, then release and continue for 5-10 repetitions.

Degenerative Disc Disease:

Degenerative disc disease is a condition that causes the discs in the spine to break down over time, resulting to pain and stiffness. Pilates routines that focus on increasing strength in the core and lower back can help relieve discomfort and increase mobility. Some examples of modified Pilates exercises for degenerative disc degeneration include the pelvic tilt and the spinal extension.

Pelvic Tilt:

Lay on your back with your legs bent and your feet flat on the ground. Inhale, then exhale as you gradually tilt your pelvis towards your belly button, flattening your lower back into the ground. Hold for 2-3 seconds, then release and continue for 10-15 repetitions.

Spinal Extension:

Lay on your stomach with your hands at your shoulders and your elbows bent. Inhale, then exhale as you lift your chest off the ground, keeping your elbows close to your sides. Hold for 2-3 seconds, then release and continue for 5-10 repetitions.

When participating in Pilates, seniors with back discomfort should also be conscious of their posture and alignment. Good posture can help prevent the risk of additional injury and enhance overall mobility. Seniors with back discomfort should attempt to maintain a neutral spine, use their core muscles, and avoid curving their shoulders or upper back.

Advanced Exercises (Optional)

Roll-Up

The Roll-Up is a popular Pilates exercise that works the core muscles and helps to develop flexibility in the spine. It is a hard exercise that requires a certain level of strength and movement. While it is normally considered an intermediate to advanced exercise, adaptations can be made to suit seniors with common difficulties such as weak abdominal muscles, tight hamstrings, and limited spine mobility.

Here are some adapted Pilates movements for seniors with these typical issues:

Weak abdominal muscles: Weak abdominal muscles might make it difficult to lift the torso off the ground during the Roll-Up exercise. Adjustments can be made to target the abdominal muscles and increase strength in this area.

Half Roll-Up: Lay down with your knees bent and your feet on the ground. Put your hands behind your head and lift your head and shoulders off the ground, curling your chin towards your chest. Hold for a few seconds, then release and repeat for 10-15 times.

Tight Hamstrings: Tight hamstrings might make it difficult to maintain the legs straight during the Roll-Up exercise. Adjustments can be made to accommodate tight hamstrings and still stimulate the core muscles.

Bent-Knee Roll-Up: Lay down on your back with your knees bent and your feet on the ground. Raise your arms towards the ceiling and lift your head and shoulders off the ground. As you drop your torso back down, bend your knees towards your chest. Repeat for 10-15 repetitions.

Reduced spine mobility: Restricted spine mobility can make it difficult to lift the torso off the ground during the Roll-Up exercise. Adjustments can be made to aid promote spine mobility and still engage the core muscles.

Seated Roll-Up: Sit on the ground with your legs straight out in front of you. Raise your arms towards the ceiling and roll your spine forward, reaching towards your toes. Gently roll back up to a seated position. Repeat for 10-15 repetitions.

It is crucial for seniors to work with a trained Pilates instructor and speak with a healthcare physician before attempting advanced Pilates exercises. Adjustments should be made as needed to fit individual needs and constraints.

In conclusion, the Roll-Up is an advanced Pilates exercise that focuses the core muscles and increases spine flexibility. Adjustments can be made to assist seniors with weak abdominal muscles, tight hamstrings, and limited spine movement. Engaging with a competent Pilates instructor and talking with a healthcare physician are crucial stages in building a safe and successful workout program for seniors.

Teaser

The Teaser is a tough and advanced Pilates exercise that involves a great level of strength, stability, and flexibility. It is a full-body workout that focuses the abdominal muscles, hip flexors, and back muscles. While it is normally considered an advanced exercise, adaptations can be made to suit seniors with common difficulties such as weak abdominal muscles, limited hip mobility, and balance issues.

Here are some adapted Pilates movements for seniors with these typical issues:

Weak abdominal muscles: Weak abdominal muscles can make it harder to lift the torso off the ground during the Teaser exercise. Adjustments can be made to target the abdominal muscles and increase strength in this area.

Half Teaser: Sit on the ground with your legs straight out in front of you. Raise your arms towards the ceiling and lift your head and shoulders off the ground. As you elevate your torso off the ground, bend your knees towards your chest. Hold for sometime, release and then repeat for 10-15 times.

Reduced hip mobility: Restricted hip mobility can make it difficult to lift the legs off the ground during the Teaser exercise. Adjustments can be made to accommodate limited hip movement and yet stimulate the core muscles.

Single-Leg Teaser: Lay on your back with your knees bent and your feet flat on the ground. Raise one leg off the ground and reach your opposite arm towards your foot. Utilize your core muscles to lift your torso off the ground and reach your hand towards your foot. Hold for a few seconds, then release and repeat on the other side for 10-15 repetitions.

Balancing difficulties: Balance issues can make it harder to maintain the right form during the Teaser exercise. Adjustments can be made to aid increase balance and stability.

Seated Teaser: Sit on the ground with your legs bent and your feet flat on the ground. Raise your arms towards the ceiling and lean back, using your core muscles to maintain balance. Raise one leg off the ground and hold for a few seconds, then release and repeat on the other side for 10-15 repetitions.

It is crucial for seniors to work with a trained Pilates instructor and speak with a healthcare physician before attempting advanced Pilates exercises. Adjustments should be made as needed to fit individual needs and constraints.

Swan

The Swan is a complex Pilates exercise that works the back, shoulders, arms, and core muscles. It entails raising the upper body off the ground while keeping the spine long and neutral. While this exercise can be difficult for seniors, it can be modified to meet typical concerns such as limited spinal movement, weak back muscles, and shoulder soreness.

The Swan is a wonderful senior exercise since it works numerous muscle groups and can improve posture, strength, and flexibility. Prior to attempting the Swan, seniors should practice fundamental Pilates movements that focus on core strength and spinal mobility.

The Swan exercise is divided into numerous separate motions. First, the senior positions themselves on their stomach, arms at their sides. They then contract their abdominal muscles and elevate their torso off the ground, maintaining a long and neutral neck and spine. They lift by drawing their shoulder blades down and back, utilizing the upper back and shoulder muscles.

When attempting the Swan exercise, elders may encounter a number of frequent problems. Common symptoms include restricted spinal motion, weakened back muscles, and shoulder pain. The exercise can be modified to meet these limitations and allow seniors to perform the Swan safely and effectively.

Spinal Mobility Issues

When performing the Swan exercise, limited spinal motion can make it difficult to lift the torso off the ground. Back muscles can be targeted and spinal mobility can be improved with modifications.

Sit on a chair with your feet flat on the ground and your hands resting on your thighs as a seated Swan. Draw your shoulder blades down and lift up your chest. Exhale and lean forward, keeping your chest elevated and your shoulder blades down and back. Hold for a few seconds before releasing and repeating for 10-15 times.

Spinal Extension with a Foam Roller: Lay on your back and place a foam roller between your shoulder blades. Lift your chest off the foam roller with your hands behind your head, maintaining your neck long and neutral. Hold for a few seconds before releasing and repeating for 10-15 times.

Muscular Weakness in the Back

Weak back muscles can make maintaining appropriate form during the Swan exercise challenging. Back muscles can be targeted and strengthened by making modifications.

Prone Arm Lifts: Lay on your stomach and extend your arms in front of you. Raise your arms above your head, keeping your shoulder blades down and back. Hold for a few seconds before releasing and repeating for 10-15 times.

Stability Ball Back Extension: Lay on a stability ball with your feet flat on the ground and your hands behind your head. Exhale while lengthening your spine and lifting your chest off the ball, maintaining your neck long and neutral. Hold for a few seconds before releasing and repeating for 10-15 times.

Shoulder Ache

Shoulder pain might make lifting the arms off the ground during the Swan exercise challenging. Back muscles can be targeted and shoulder mobility can be improved with modifications.

Stability of a Swan Lay on a stability ball, hands on the ground in front of you. Step forward with your hands until your hips are on the ball and your arms are completely extended. Draw your shoulder blades down and lift your chest. Inhale to stretch your spine, exhale to elevate your chest off the ball while keeping your arms straight. Hold for a few seconds before releasing and repeating for 10-15 times.

Swan on a Foam Roller: Lay on your stomach and place a foam roller under your sternum. Lift your chest off the foam roller with your hands behind your head, maintaining your neck long and neutral. Hold for a few seconds before releasing and repeating for 10-15 times.

Seniors can benefit from incorporating the Swan exercise into their Pilates regimen. It can aid in the improvement of posture, the strengthening of back muscles, and the expansion of spinal mobility. Nonetheless, seniors should work with a competent Pilates instructor to ensure that the exercise is done safely and successfully.

<u>The following are some hints for executing the Swan exercise</u>:

-Before attempting the Swan, begin with basic Pilates movements to increase core strength and spinal mobility.

-Throughout the exercise, keep your spine long and neutral.

-Pull the shoulder blades down and back to engage the upper back and shoulder muscles.

-Avoid raising the head too high, as this might put strain on the neck.

-Modifications can be used to address common difficulties such limited spinal movement, weak back muscles, and shoulder pain.

-To ensure good form and technique, work with a competent Pilates instructor.

In conclusion, the Swan exercise is an advanced Pilates exercise that works the muscles of the back, shoulders, arms, and core. Seniors can benefit from include this exercise in their Pilates regimen, but changes may be required to meet typical concerns such limited spinal mobility, weak back muscles, and shoulder pain. Engaging with a certified Pilates instructor can help elders perform the exercise safely and successfully.

Saw

The Saw exercise is a more advanced Pilates exercise that works the back, hips, and core muscles. It is an excellent exercise for increasing spine rotation and general flexibility. However, elders may experience common difficulties such as limited spinal mobility, stiff hips, and weak core muscles, which can make performing the Saw exercise safely and efficiently challenging. In this sub chapter, we will describe how to perform the Saw exercise with modified workouts for typical concerns on Pilates for seniors.

How to Carry Out the Saw Workout

Begin the Saw exercise by sitting tall on a mat, legs straight out in front of you, hip-width apart. Stretch your arms out to the sides, with your palm facing the floor. Inhale and turn your torso to the right, bringing your left hand to your right foot. Exhale as you twist your torso to the right and reach your right arm behind you. Maintain a forward look and sturdy hips. Inhale and return to the beginning position, then do the opposite side. Attempt 10-15 repetitions.

Benefit of Modified Saw Exercises

Spinal Mobility Issues

Seniors with poor spinal mobility may struggle to fully rotate their torso during the Saw exercise. Begin by performing a mild spinal twist while seated to accommodate this. Sit upright on a mat, your legs straight out in front of you, hip-width apart. Stretch your arms out to the sides, palms down. Inhale and turn to the right, bringing your left hand toward your right knee. Exhale and rotate to the right a little more, maintaining your gaze forward and your hips stable. Inhale and return to the beginning position, then do the opposite side. Attempt 10-15 repetitions.

Tight Hips

Seniors with tight hips may struggle to keep their pelvis stable when executing the Saw exercise. Begin by doing a seated forward fold while sitting on a folded towel or blanket. Sit upright on a mat, your legs straight out in front of you, hip-width apart. Exhale and raise your arms overhead. Exhale and fold forward from the hips, bringing your arms toward the ground. Inhale and return to the beginning posture after 5-10 breaths. Repeat 3-5 times more.

Weak Core Muscles

Seniors with weak core muscles may struggle to maintain good form and alignment throughout the Saw exercise. Begin by practicing a modified version of the Saw exercise with a Pilates ring or ball for support. Sit upright on a mat, your legs straight out in front of you, hip-width apart. With your arms straight out in front of you, hold the Pilates ring or ball between your hands. Inhale and turn your torso to the right, aiming for the ring or ball near your right foot. Exhale and rotate to the right a little more, maintaining your gaze forward and your hips stable. Inhale and return to the beginning position, then do the opposite side. Attempt 10-15 repetitions.

Adding the Saw exercise into a Pilates regimen can be good for elders. It can assist improve spinal rotation, promote flexibility, and strengthen back, hip, and core muscles. Nonetheless, seniors should work with a competent Pilates instructor to ensure that the exercise is done safely and successfully.

<u>Here are some pointers for conducting the Saw exercise</u>:

-Before attempting the Saw, begin with fundamental Pilates movements to increase core strength and spinal mobility.

-Throughout the exercise, keep your spine long and neutral.

-Use your core muscles to stabilize your pelvis and support your spine.

-Maintain a forward gaze and relaxed shoulders.

-Increase the number of repetitions and work on extending your range of motion as you feel more comfortable with the Saw exercise.

CHAPTER 5:

Pilates Equipment for Seniors

For seniors over the age of 60, Pilates can be a highly effective form of exercise to maintain fitness, improve posture, and prevent injuries. In this chapter, we will introduce the many forms of Pilates equipment suitable for seniors over 60.

The Reformer

The Pilates Reformer is possibly the most well-known piece of Pilates equipment. It comprises of a frame with a sliding carriage, foot bar, and variable resistance springs. The Reformer delivers a full-body workout, and it can be adjusted to fit the demands of each unique user. For seniors over 60, the Reformer can be a highly effective tool to enhance posture, balance, and overall fitness.

The Reformer provides a low-impact workout that is soft on the joints, making it great for seniors who may be battling with joint discomfort or other ailments. The sliding carriage of the Reformer enables for smooth, regulated movements, making it easier for elders to retain appropriate form while exercising. The foot bar and resistance springs provide variable levels of resistance, allowing users to progress their workouts as they become stronger and more fit.

One of the primary benefits of the Reformer is its capacity to develop core strength. The sliding carriage and resistance springs give a dynamic workout that targets the core muscles during the whole workout. For seniors over 60, this can be particularly effective in preventing falls and keeping good balance.

The Cadillac

The Pilates Cadillac, also known as the Trapeze Table, is another piece of equipment that is suitable for seniors over 60. It comprises of a frame with an elevated platform and a system of overhead bars and straps. The Cadillac is a full-body workout that focuses on improving flexibility, balance, and core strength.

The raised platform of the Cadillac provides a secure and sturdy surface for elders to undertake activities that require balance and stability. The overhead bars and straps can be used to conduct a number of workouts that target different muscular areas, including the arms, legs, and core. The Cadillac also includes a number of accessories, such as springs, bars, and straps, which can be used to adjust exercises and give varied levels of resistance.

For seniors, the Cadillac might be particularly effective in developing flexibility. The overhead bars and straps enable for stretching exercises that can assist to increase range of motion and alleviate muscular tightness. The Cadillac can also be used to conduct workouts that target the lower back and hips, which can help to reduce pain and improve general mobility.

The Wunda Chair

The Wunda Chair is a compact piece of Pilates equipment that is excellent for seniors over 60 who may be struggling with limited mobility or space constraints. It comprises of a small, elevated platform with a spring-loaded pedal and a set of handles. The Wunda Chair provides a low-impact workout that is soft on the joints, making it excellent for seniors who may be battling with joint discomfort or other ailments.

The spring-loaded pedal of the Wunda Chair provides resistance that may be adjusted to fit the demands of each unique user. The handles can be utilized to do a number of workouts that target different muscular areas, including the arms, legs, and core. The tiny design of the Wunda Chair makes it easy to store and use in small locations, such as a home gym or living room.

For seniors over 60, the Wunda Chair can be particularly effective in strengthening core strength and balance. The spring-loaded pedal offers resistance that engages the core muscles during the entire workout. The handles can also be utilized to execute exercises that target the upper body, which can help to enhance general strength and posture.

The Ladder Barrel

The Ladder Barrel is a piece of Pilates equipment that is perfect for seniors over 60 who may be battling with back pain or other difficulties linked to spinal health. It consists of a barrel-shaped frame with a set of rungs and a padded surface. The Ladder Barrel delivers a low-impact workout that focuses on improving flexibility, posture, and overall spinal health.

The rungs of the Ladder Barrel can be utilized to do a variety of exercises that target different muscular areas, including the back, legs, and core. The padded surface provides a pleasant and supportive surface for seniors to conduct exercises that require lying down or sitting. The Ladder Barrel may also be altered to suit the demands of each individual user, making it a versatile piece of equipment for seniors over 60.

For adults over 60, the Ladder Barrel can be very effective in promoting spinal health. The movements performed on the Ladder Barrel can assist to stretch and strengthen the muscles and ligaments surrounding the spine, which can help to reduce discomfort and improve overall mobility. The Ladder Barrel can also be used to perform workouts that target the core muscles, which can assist to improve posture and prevent falls.

The Pilates Mat

While not strictly a piece of Pilates equipment, the Pilates Mat is a crucial tool for seniors over 60 who are trying to enhance their fitness and overall health. The Pilates Mat delivers a low-impact workout that focuses on building core strength, flexibility, and general body alignment.

The Pilates Mat can be used to do a range of exercises that target different muscular areas, including the core, arms, legs, and back. The exercises may be changed to fit the demands of each individual user, making the Pilates Mat a versatile tool for seniors over 60. The Pilates Mat can also be used in conjunction with other Pilates equipment, such as the Reformer or Cadillac, to create a more comprehensive workout.

The Pilates Mat can be very effective in improving posture and preventing falls. The movements performed on the Pilates Mat can assist to strengthen the core muscles, which are vital for maintaining good balance and stability. The Pilates Mat can also be used to conduct exercises that target the lower back and hips, which can assist to reduce discomfort and improve overall mobility.

Using the reformer

The Reformer is a bed-like frame with a sliding carriage that is coupled to springs and pulleys. The Reformer is a low-impact workout that focuses on building flexibility, balance, and overall strength. In this post, we will examine how seniors over 60 can utilize the Reformer equipment to improve their fitness and overall health.

Advantages of Using the Reformer Equipment for Seniors Over 60

The Reformer provides various benefits for elders over 60. Some of the primary benefits include:

Low-Impact Workout: The Reformer gives a low-impact workout that is gentle on the joints. This makes it a perfect kind of exercise for seniors over 60 who may be battling with arthritis or other joint-related concerns.

Increased Flexibility: The Reformer gives a broad range of motion that can aid to enhance flexibility and mobility. The movements performed on the Reformer can assist to stretch and strengthen the muscles, which can enhance overall joint health.

Increased Core Strength: The Reformer delivers an effective workout for the core muscles, which are vital for maintaining good posture, balance, and stability. A strong core can also assist to reduce falls, which can be a serious issue for seniors over 60.

Better Balance: The Reformer gives a workout that targets the muscles responsible for balance and stability. This can help to improve general balance, which can also help to prevent falls.

Better Posture: The Reformer gives a workout that targets the muscles necessary for proper posture. This can assist to improve general body alignment and lessen the risk of back pain.

<u>How to Utilize the Reformer Equipment for Elderly Over 60</u>

The Reformer can be used to execute a number of exercises that target different muscle groups. Here are some recommendations on how seniors over 60 can use the

Reformer equipment to improve their fitness and overall health:

Start Slowly: It is crucial to start slowly when utilizing the Reformer. Seniors over 60 should begin with basic workouts and progressively build up to more strenuous routines.

Utilize the Springs to Change Resistance: The springs on the Reformer can be modified to offer more or less resistance. Seniors over 60 should start with lighter resistance and progressively increase as they become stronger.

Employ the Foot Bar for Stability: The foot bar on the Reformer can be utilized for stability during workouts that require lying down or sitting. Seniors over 60 can use the foot bar to support their feet and maintain good posture during workouts.

Employ the Straps for Assistance: The straps on the Reformer can be used for aid during workouts that require additional strength or flexibility. Seniors over 60 can use the straps to help them accomplish exercises that may be too tough without assistance.

Emphasis on Breathing: Breathing is a key aspect of Pilates. Adults over 60 should focus on breathing deeply and gently during their workout. This can help to increase general relaxation and reduce tension.

Exercises to Do on the Reformer Equipment

The Reformer can be used to execute a number of exercises that target different muscle groups. Here are some workouts that are good for adults;

Footwork: Footwork is a simple workout that can help to enhance total leg strength and flexibility. Seniors over 60 can practice footwork by lying on their back with their feet on the foot bar. Kids can then push the carriage away from their body with their feet and then bring it back in.

Hundred: Hundred is an exercise that emphasizes the core muscles. Seniors over 60 can execute Hundred by lying on their back with their legs in a tabletop position and their arms extended towards the ceiling. They can then pump their arms up and down while maintaining a solid core.

Leg Circles: Leg circles are an exercise that focuses the hip flexors and the core muscles. Seniors over 60 can execute leg circles by lying on their back with their legs extended towards the ceiling. They can then rotate their legs in a circular manner while maintaining a stable core.

Arm Circles: Arm circles are an exercise that focuses the shoulder muscles and the core muscles. Seniors over 60 can execute arm circles by lying on their back with their arms extended towards the ceiling. They can then rotate their arms in a circular manner while maintaining a stable core.

Side Leg Series: Side leg series is an exercise that targets the outer hip muscles and the core muscles. Seniors over 60 can execute side leg series by lying on their side with their legs stretched towards the foot bar. They can then lift and drop their top leg while maintaining a solid core.

Using the chair

The chair delivers a low-impact workout that focuses on improving flexibility, balance, and overall strength. In this post, we will examine how seniors over 60 can use the chair equipment to improve their fitness and overall health.

Advantages of Utilizing the Chair Equipment for Seniors Over 60

The chair provides various benefits for people over 60. Some of the primary benefits include:

Low-Impact Workout: The chair gives a low-impact workout that is mild on the joints. This makes it a perfect kind of exercise for seniors over 60 who may be battling with arthritis or other joint-related concerns.

Increased Flexibility: The chair gives a full range of motion that can aid to enhance flexibility and mobility. The exercises performed on the chair can assist to stretch and strengthen the muscles, which can enhance overall joint health.

Increased Core Strength: The chair provides an effective workout for the core muscles, which are necessary for maintaining good posture, balance, and stability. A strong core can also assist to reduce falls, which can be a serious issue for seniors over 60.

Better Balance: The chair delivers a workout that targets the muscles responsible for balance and stability. This can help to improve general balance, which can also help to prevent falls.

Better Posture: The chair gives a workout that targets the muscles responsible for proper posture. This can assist to improve general body alignment and lessen the risk of back pain.

How to Utilize the Chair Equipment for Seniors

The chair may be used to execute a number of workouts that target different muscle areas. Here are some recommendations on how seniors over 60 can use the chair equipment to improve their fitness and general health:

Start Slowly: It is recommended to start slowly when utilizing the chair. Seniors over 60 should begin with basic workouts and progressively build up to more strenuous routines.

Employ the Chair for Support: The chair can be utilized for support during exercises that involve standing or balancing. Seniors over 60 can use the chair to support their weight and maintain good posture during workouts.

Employ the Chair for Resistance: The chair can be used to offer resistance during workouts that demand more strength or flexibility. Seniors over 60 can utilize the chair to help them accomplish exercises that may be too tough without assistance.

Emphasis on Breathing: Breathing is a key aspect of Pilates. Adults over 60 should focus on breathing deeply and gently during their workout. This can help to increase general relaxation and reduce tension.

Exercises to Perform on the Chair Equipment for Seniors

The chair may be used to execute a number of workouts that target different muscle areas. Here are some workouts that are good for adults over 60:

Seated Leg Lifts: Seated leg lifts are an exercise that targets the core muscles and the leg muscles. Seniors over 60 can perform seated leg lifts by sitting on the chair with their feet flat on the ground. They can then elevate one leg at a time while keeping a steady core.

Standing Leg Lifts: Standing leg lifts are an exercise that focuses the leg muscles and the core muscles. Seniors over 60 can perform standing leg lifts by standing behind the chair with their hands resting on the back of the chair. They can then elevate one leg at a time while keeping a steady core.

Chair Squats: Chair squats are an exercise that focuses the leg muscles and the core muscles. Seniors over 60 can perform chair squats by standing in front of the chair with their feet shoulder-width apart. They can then sit back into the chair as if they were going to sit down, and then stand back up while maintaining good posture.

Arm Circles: Arm circles are an exercise that focuses the shoulder muscles and the core muscles. Seniors over 60 can conduct arm circles by sitting on the chair with their arms extended towards the ceiling. They can then rotate their arms in a circular manner while maintaining a stable core.

Seated Twist: Sitting twist is an exercise that focuses the core muscles and the back muscles. Seniors over 60 can execute seated twist by sitting on the chair with their feet flat on the ground. They can then twist their upper body to the left and then to the right while keeping a solid core.

Single-Leg Raises: Single-leg rises are an exercise that focuses the leg muscles and the core muscles. Seniors over 60 can perform single-leg lifts by sitting on the chair with their feet flat on the ground. They can then elevate one leg at a time while keeping a steady core.

Side-Leg Lifts: Side-leg lifts are an exercise that targets the outer hip muscles and the core muscles. Seniors over 60 can perform side-leg lifts by standing behind the chair with their hands resting on the back of the chair. They can then lift one leg out to the side while keeping a solid core.

Using the Cadillac

Pilates equipment, such as the Cadillac, can allow adults over 60 to undertake a number of exercises that target different muscle regions. In this essay, we will discuss how seniors over 60 can use the Cadillac equipment to improve their general health and well-being.

What is the Cadillac?

The Cadillac is a piece of Pilates equipment that comprises of a metal frame with numerous bars and straps attached to it. It was originally devised by Joseph Pilates to help wounded dancers and athletes recuperate from their ailments. The Cadillac is also known as the Trapeze Table since it has a trapeze attached to it that may be used for a variety of workouts.

Utilizing the Cadillac for Seniors

The Cadillac is an ideal piece of equipment for seniors over 60 since it gives a low-impact workout that can assist to improve flexibility, balance, and general strength. Here are some activities that seniors over 60 can perform on the Cadillac:

Leg Springs: Leg springs are an exercise that focuses the leg muscles and the core muscles. Seniors over 60 can practice leg springs by lying on their back on the Cadillac with their feet in the straps. They can then lift their legs up and down while maintaining a solid core.

Arm Springs: Arm springs are an exercise that focuses the arm muscles and the core muscles. Seniors over 60 can practice arm springs by sitting on the Cadillac with their arms in the straps. They can then push their arms out and in while maintaining a solid core.

Roll-Downs: Roll-downs are an exercise that focuses the core muscles and the back muscles. Seniors over 60 can perform roll-downs by sitting on the Cadillac with their legs extended towards the trapeze. They can then roll down through their spine and touch their toes to the trapeze while maintaining a steady core.

Standing Leg Springs: Standing leg springs are an exercise that focuses the leg muscles and the core muscles. Seniors over 60 can execute standing leg springs by standing on the Cadillac with one foot in the strap. They can then lift their leg up and down while maintaining a solid core.

Bridging: Bridging is an exercise that focuses the core muscles and the back muscles. Seniors over 60 can do bridging by lying on their back on the Cadillac with their feet on the trapeze. They can then lift their hips up towards the ceiling while maintaining a steady core.

Side-Leg Springs: Side-leg springs are an activity that targets the outer hip muscles and the core muscles. Seniors over 60 can practice side-leg springs by lying on their side on the Cadillac with their legs in the straps. They can then lift their top leg up and down while maintaining a solid core.

Pull-Ups: Pull-ups are an activity that stimulates the arm muscles and the core muscles. Seniors over 60 can execute pull-ups by standing on the Cadillac with their hands in the straps. They can then bring their body up towards the straps while keeping a steady core.

Advantages of Using the Cadillac for Seniors

There are several perks to using the Cadillac for seniors over 60. Here are some of the primary benefits:

Increases Flexibility: The Cadillac can help seniors over 60 to enhance their flexibility by delivering a low-impact workout that targets different muscle areas.

Builds Core Strength: The Cadillac can enable seniors over 60 to increase their core strength by giving a variety of exercises that target the core muscles.

Enhances Balance: The Cadillac can help seniors over 60 to strengthen their balance by delivering exercises that demand stability and control.

Low-Impact: The Cadillac is a low-impact workout that is suited for seniors over 60 who may have joint pain or other health concerns.

Increases Posture: The Cadillac can help seniors over 60 to enhance their posture by giving exercises that target the back and core muscles.

Improves Strength: The Cadillac can enable seniors over 60 to increase their overall strength by giving a variety of exercises that target different muscle regions.

Reduces Pain: The Cadillac can help seniors over 60 to lessen pain by delivering a low-impact workout that targets certain muscle regions that may be causing pain or discomfort.

Tips for staying motivated and committed to your Pilates practice

Staying motivated and committed to your Pilates practice as a senior can sometimes be challenging. However, by following these tips, you can stay motivated and committed to your Pilates practice:

Set Realistic Goals

Setting realistic goals for yourself is essential to staying motivated and committed to your Pilates practice. It's important to set goals that are achievable and measurable, such as practicing Pilates for 30 minutes three times a week. As you achieve your goals, you can gradually increase the frequency and duration of your Pilates practice.

Make it Fun

Making your Pilates practice fun can help you to stay motivated and committed. Consider incorporating props, such as resistance bands or Pilates balls, into your practice, or trying new exercises or variations of familiar exercises. You can also consider practicing Pilates in different locations, such as outside or in a new room in your home.

Track Your Progress

Tracking your progress can help you to stay motivated and committed to your Pilates practice. Consider keeping a journal or using a Pilates app to track your progress and set reminders for your practice sessions. Seeing your progress over time can help you to stay motivated and committed to your Pilates practice.

Find an Accountability Partner

Having an accountability partner can help you to stay motivated and committed to your Pilates practice. Consider finding a friend or family member to practice Pilates with, or join a Pilates class where you can connect with other Pilates enthusiasts. Having someone to share your progress with and to hold you accountable can help you to stay motivated and committed.

Practice Mindfulness

Practicing mindfulness during your Pilates practice can help you to stay present and engaged, which can help you to stay motivated and committed. Focus on your breath and the movements of your body during your Pilates practice, and try to be present in the moment. Practicing mindfulness can also help to reduce stress and improve mental clarity.

Mix It Up

Mixing up your Pilates routine can help you to stay motivated and committed. Consider trying new exercises or incorporating different props or modifications into your practice. This can help to challenge your body and keep your Pilates practice fresh and engaging.

Celebrate Your Progress

Celebrating your progress can help you to stay motivated and committed to your Pilates practice. Celebrate each achievement, no matter how small, and give yourself credit for the work you've done. Celebrating your progress can help to boost your confidence and motivation to continue your Pilates practice.

Find a Time that Works for You

To make Pilates a part of your daily routine, it's important to find a time that works for you. Some seniors prefer to practice Pilates in the morning to help them start their day, while others prefer to practice in the evening to help them unwind after a busy day. Choose a time that works best for you and stick to it.

Incorporate Pilates into Your Daily Activities

In addition to dedicating specific time slots for Pilates practice, you can also integrate Pilates into your daily activities. For example, you can practice breathing exercises while you are waiting in line at the grocery store or do some gentle stretches while you are watching TV.

Use Pilates Props

Pilates props, such as resistance bands, Pilates balls, and foam rollers, can help to add variety and challenge to your Pilates practice. Using props can also make Pilates more fun and enjoyable. Incorporate props into your Pilates practice as you become more comfortable with the exercises.

Mindfulness and Stress Management

Mindfulness is a method that has been increasingly popular in recent years as an aid for stress management and overall well-being. Pilates is an exercise method that can combine mindfulness techniques to boost its advantages for seniors over 60. Mindfulness can be defined as the discipline of being present in the moment, fully involved in whatever is happening without judgment or distraction. Integrating mindfulness into a Pilates practice can enable seniors to reduce stress, improve focus and concentration, and promote general well-being.

These are some ways that mindfulness can be used into Pilates for seniors over 60 to assist stress management:

Concentrate on breath

One of the most important parts of mindfulness is focusing on breath. In Pilates, breath work is a crucial component of the exercises. Teaching seniors to focus on their breath throughout each movement can enable them to become more present in the moment and shut out any distractions or worries.

Tune into body Sensations

Mindfulness means tuning into the sensations of the body without judgment. In Pilates, seniors can be taught to tune into the feelings of each movement and become more aware of how their body is feeling. This can enable individuals to become more in tune with their body and minimize stress by being more present in the moment.

Incorporate Meditation

Meditation is a technique that is widely utilized in mindfulness practice. Seniors can be encouraged to take a few moments at the beginning or finish of their Pilates practice to meditate. This can enable individuals to quiet the mind, reduce tension, and promote general well-being.

Practice Gratitude

Gratitude is a vital component of mindfulness. Asking seniors to spend a few moments at the end of their Pilates exercise to reflect on what they are grateful for will enable them to create a more positive mentality and reduce stress.

Engage the Senses

Engaging the senses is another approach to incorporate mindfulness into Pilates practice. Seniors can be encouraged to focus on the sights, sounds, and sensations of their environment throughout their practice. This can allow individuals to become more present in the moment and minimize stress.

Incorporate Affirmations

Affirmations are uplifting remarks that can be used to build a positive mindset. Seniors can be encouraged to include affirmations into their Pilates practice to help reduce stress and increase general well-being. This can involve repeating encouraging phrases to themselves during their practice or using visual signals such as post-it notes with positive affirmations inscribed on them.

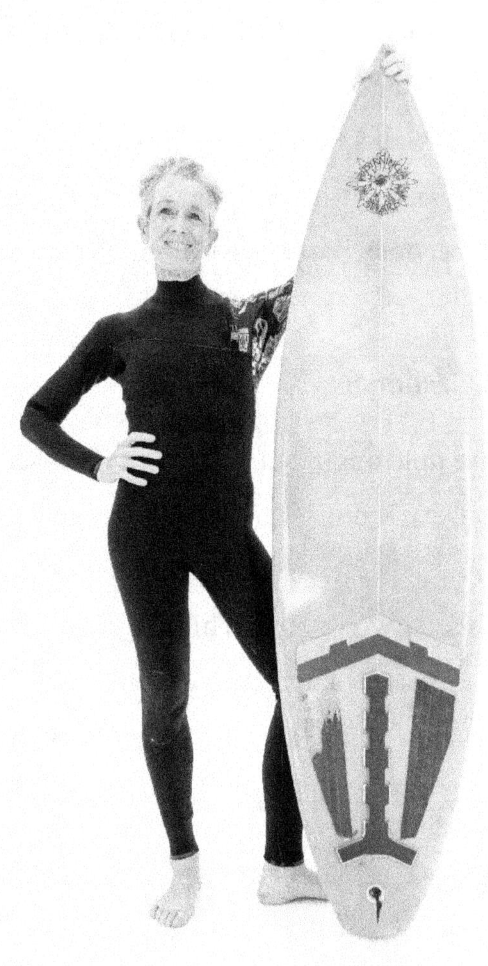

Conclusion

In conclusion, Pilates is a low-impact exercise form that can offer numerous benefits for seniors. Pilates can help to improve strength, flexibility, balance, and posture, while also promoting mind-body wellness and stress management. The use of Pilates equipment, such as the reformer, chair, and Cadillac, can offer additional benefits and provide modifications for seniors with varying levels of ability.

It is important for seniors to take safety precautions when practicing Pilates, including consulting with a healthcare provider, starting with a beginner class, using appropriate equipment, using proper form and technique, avoiding over-exertion, staying hydrated, and wearing appropriate clothing. By taking these precautions, seniors can reduce the risk of injury and maximize the benefits of their Pilates practice.

Overall, Pilates is a great exercise form for seniors who are looking to improve their overall health and wellness. With its focus on mindful movement, Pilates can help seniors stay active and engaged in their physical fitness, while also promoting mental and emotional well-being. By incorporating Pilates into their daily routine, seniors can stay strong, flexible, and healthy, while also enjoying the many benefits of this popular exercise form.

* 9 7 9 8 3 7 9 2 7 5 1 5 0 *